Symptoms in the Pharmacy

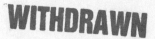

Symptoms in the Pharmacy

A Guide to the Management of Common Illness

ALISON BLENKINSOPP

BPharm, MRPharmS, PhD
Director of Education and Research
Department of Medicines Management
Keele University

AND

PAUL PAXTON

MB, ChB, MRCGP, DRCOG
General Practitioner, Cambridge

THIRD EDITION

**Blackwell
Science**

© 1989, 1995, 1998 by
Blackwell Science Ltd
Editorial Offices:
Osney Mead, Oxford OX2 0EL
25 John Street, London WC1N 2BL
23 Ainslie Place, Edinburgh EH3 6AJ
350 Main Street, Malden
  MA 02148 5018, USA
54 University Street, Carlton
  Victoria 3053, Australia
10, rue Casimir Delavigne
  75006 Paris, France

Other Editorial Offices:

Blackwell Wissenschafts-Verlag GmbH
Kurfürstendamm 57
10707 Berlin, Germany

Blackwell Science KK
MG Kodenmacho Building
7–10 Kodenmacho Nihombashi
Chuo-ku, Tokyo 104, Japan

First published 1989
Reprinted 1990, 1992, 1993
Spanish translation 1992
Japanese translation 1993
Second edition 1995
Reprinted 1996, 1997
Third edition 1998
Reprinted 1998

Set by Setrite Typesetters, Hong Kong
Printed and bound in Great Britain by
MPG Books Ltd, Bodmin, Cornwall

The Blackwell Science logo is a
trade mark of Blackwell Science Ltd,
registered at the United Kingdom
Trade Marks Registry

DISTRIBUTORS

Marston Book Services Ltd
PO Box 269
Abingdon
Oxon OX14 4YN
(*Orders:* Tel: 01235 465500
        Fax: 01235 465555)

USA
Blackwell Science, Inc.
Commerce Place
350 Main Street
Malden, MA 02148 5018
(*Orders:* Tel: 800 759 6102
                781 388 8250
        Fax: 781 388 8255)

Canada
Login Brothers Book Company
324 Saulteaux Crescent
Winnipeg, Manitoba R3J 3T2
(*Orders:* Tel: 204 224-4068)

Australia
Blackwell Science Pty Ltd
54 University Street
Carlton, Victoria 3053
(*Orders:* Tel: 03 9347 0300
        Fax: 03 9347 5001)

A catalogue record for this title
is available from the British Library

ISBN 0–632–04941–3

For further information on Blackwell Science,
visit our website:
www.blackwell-science.com

Contents

Preface to the third edition

It is now 10 years since we wrote the first edition of this book in 1988. Since then the range of treatments which pharmacists can recommend has been greatly increased by the movement of many medicines from the 'prescription only medicine' (POM) category to the 'pharmacy medicine' (P) category. These changes mean that pharmacists at all stages of their career need practical information to help them in dealing with new areas of patient care and ensuring their knowledge is up to date.

The second edition of this book appeared in 1994 and, in addition to general updating, included new chapters on the treatment of mouth ulcers and vaginal thrush in response to POM to P moves of vaginal imidazoles and acyclovir.

In this, the third edition, there are new sections on irritable bowel syndrome, dandruff and hair loss to provide further guidance for pharmacists following key POM to P changes in these areas and also new sections on insomnia and psoriasis. Each of the existing chapters has been updated and many extensively rewritten to take account of the availability of new medicines, changes in approaches to treatment (for example, in head lice and scabies) and the emergence of new evidence on effectiveness, interactions and adverse effects.

With the increasing emphasis on the pharmacist's role as a 'first port of call' in response to symptoms, the need for effective communication and interpersonal skills remains paramount. Appropriate techniques for gathering information from patients/clients to meet the needs of patient safety in a way that is acceptable to the public have been highlighted. Therefore we have again revised the introductory chapter to give further guidance on questioning and listening skills.

We have received many positive letters and comments from pharmacists (undergraduate students, pre-registration trainees and practising pharmacists) all over the world following the earlier editions of the book and have tried to act on our readers' suggestions. We would like to thank all the pharmacists who contributed in this way and hope that this new edition of the book will meet the needs they have helped us to identify.

Alison Blenkinsopp
Paul Paxton

Introduction: How to use this book

Every working day, the community pharmacist is asked by members of the public for advice about symptoms. For the average community pharmacist a minimum of 10 such requests will be received each day; for some the figure is far higher. Another group of pharmacy customers present by asking to purchase a named product. Such requests appear to be increasing as more advertising is direct to the public.

The pharmacist is increasingly seen as a source of accessible, informed and reliable health advice. Each year, millions of pounds' worth of over-the-counter (OTC) medicines are purchased, and the community pharmacist is in an excellent position to give advice about their correct use.

The pharmacist's role in responding to symptoms and overseeing the sale of OTC medicines is substantial and requires a mix of knowledge and skills in the area of diseases and their treatment. Key skills are:

differentiation between minor and more serious symptoms

listening skills

questioning skills

treatment choices based on evidence of effectiveness

the ability to pass these skills on by acting as a role model for other pharmacy staff.

The Royal Pharmaceutical Society (RPSGB) has, since January 1995, required all community pharmacies to have a written protocol for the sales of OTC medicines. The word protocol simply means a way of doing things and indicates the procedures to be followed in that pharmacy. Standards for the sales of OTC medicines were published in autumn 1996 and these set out the approaches to be followed in the two main situations:

request for advice about symptoms

request to purchase a named product.

As a result of the introduction of protocols, more questions are being asked of members of the public before a medicine is sold in a pharmacy. Research shows that the majority of pharmacy customers do not mind being asked such questions. An exception to this is a small number of people who wish to buy a medicine they have used before and would prefer not to be subjected to the same questions each time they ask for the product. There are two key points here for the pharmacist:

it can be helpful to briefly explain why questions are needed, and normally fewer questions are needed where a customer requests a named medicine that they have used before.

A suggested sequence to respond to a request for a named product is as follows:

ask whether the person has used the medicine before

if the answer is yes, ask if they need any further information

a quick check on whether other medicines are being taken can be useful.

If the person has not used the medicine before more questions will be needed. One option is to follow the sequence for responding to advice about symptoms (see below). It can be useful to ask how the person came to request this particular medicine, for example, have they seen an advertisement for it? Has it been recommended by a friend or family member?

Pharmacists will use their professional judgement in dealing with regular customers whom they know well and where the individual's medication history is known. The pharmacy patient medication records (PMRs) are a source of back-up information for regular customers. However, for new customers where such information is not known, more questions are likely to be needed. Responding to requests for advice about symptoms requires more information gathering.

A suggested sequence for responding to symptoms is described below:

Listening and Questioning: to obtain information about symptoms

Decision-making: is referral for a medical opinion required?

Treatment: the selection of an appropriate preparation (where needed) and advising on its use.

Outcome: telling the patient what action to take if the symptoms do not improve.

Listening

Most information required to make a decision and recommend treatment can be gleaned from just listening to the patient. The process should start with open-type questions and perhaps an explanation of why it is necessary to ask personal questions. Some patients do not yet understand why the pharmacist needs to ask questions before recommending treatment. An example might be:

Patient: 'Can you give me something for my piles?'

Pharmacist: 'I'm sure I can. To help me give the best advice though, I'd like a bit more information from you, so I need to ask a few questions. Is that OK?'

Patient: 'That's fine.'

Pharmacist: 'Could you just tell me what sort of trouble you get with your piles?'

Hopefully this will lead to a description of most of the symptoms required for the pharmacist to make an assessment. Other forms of open questions could include: 'How does that affect you? What sort of problems does it cause you?'. By carefully listening and possibly reflecting back comments made by the patient the pharmacist can get a more complete picture.

Patient: 'Well, I get spells of bleeding, and soreness. It's been going on for years.'

Pharmacist: 'You say years?'

Patient: 'Yes, on and off for twenty years since may last pregnancy. I've seen my doctor several times and had them injected, but it keeps coming back. My doctor said I'd have to have an operation but I don't want one; can you give me some suppositories to stop them bleeding?'

Pharmacist: 'Bleeding...?'

Patient: 'Yes, every time I go to the toilet blood splashes around the toilet. It's bright red.'

This form of listening can be helped by asking questions to clarify points: 'I'm not sure I quite understand when you say ...', or 'I'm not quite clear what you meant by ...'. Another useful technique is to summarize the information so far: 'I'd just like to make sure I've got it right. You tell me you've had this problem since ...'.

Once this form of information gathering has occurred there will be some facts still missing. It is now appropriate to move onto some direct questions. The areas that need to be covered are in the next section on *Questioning*. Typical closed questions would include: 'What treatment have you tried before? Do you have any other trouble with your bowels? Do you go regularly? Has there been any recent change? Do you have any allergies?'.

Questioning

Where advice about symptoms is requested the pharmacist will need to question patients about their symptoms. A structured approach to questioning will ensure that all important areas are covered. Areas of questioning are discussed in each section of this book in relation to specific symptoms. Priority questions can be summarized in an acronym—this is intended to act as a reminder of the key areas. The order of questions, their phrasing and the questioning style are individual to the pharmacist.

W   Who is the patient and what are the symptoms?

H How long have the symptoms been present?
A Action taken?
M Medication being taken?

The pharmacist must first establish the identity of the patient: the person in the pharmacy might be there on someone else's behalf. The exact nature of the symptoms should be established; patients often self-diagnose illnesses and the pharmacist must not accept such a self-diagnosis at face value.

Duration of symptoms can be an important indicator of whether referral to the doctor might be required. In general, the longer the duration the more likely the possibility of a serious rather than minor case. Most minor conditions are self-limiting and should clear up within a few days.

Any action taken by the patient should be established, including the use of any medication to treat the symptoms. About one in two patients will have tried at least one remedy before seeking the pharmacist's advice. Treatment may have consisted of OTC medicines bought from the pharmacy or elsewhere, other medicines prescribed by the doctor on this or a previous occasion, or medicines 'borrowed' from a friend or neighbour or 'found' in the medicine cabinet. Homeopathic or herbal remedies may have been used.

If the patient has used one or more apparently appropriate treatments without improvement, referral to the family doctor may be the best course of action.

The identity of any medicines taken regularly by the patient is important for two reasons: possible interactions and potential adverse reactions. Such medicines will usually be those prescribed by the doctor, but may also include OTC products. The pharmacist needs to know about all the medicines being taken by the patient because of the potential for interaction with any treatment which the pharmacist might recommend.

The community pharmacist has an increasingly important role in detecting adverse drug reactions and consideration should be given to the possibility that the patient's symptoms might be an adverse effect caused by medication. For example, whether gastric symptoms such as indigestion might be due to a non-steroidal anti-inflammatory drug (NSAID) taken on prescription, or a cough might be due to an angiotensin-converting enzyme (ACE) inhibitor being taken by the patient. Where the pharmacist suspects an adverse drug reaction to a prescribed medicine, the pharmacist should discuss with the doctor what actions should be taken (perhaps including a report to the Committee on Safety of Medicines) and the doctor may wish the patient to be referred to that treatment can be reviewed.

A second mnemonic can be used to illustrate further areas of information which might be needed. Again it is useful to stress that while mnemonics are helpful memory-joggers it is up to each pharmacist to develop their own method of questioning in a style which suits them and can be carried out conversationally with patients rather than appearing as an interrogatory checklist.

A   Age/appearance
S   Self or someone else
M   Medication (regularly taken, on prescription, or OTC)
E   Extra medicines (any tried to treat the current symptoms)
T   Time persisting
H   History
O   Other symptoms
D   Danger symptoms

Some of the areas covered by the ASMETHOD list have been discussed already. The others can now be considered.

Age and appearance

The appearance of the patient can be a useful indicator of whether a minor or more serious condition is involved. If the patient looks ill, for example, pale, clammy, flushed or grey, the pharmacist should consider referral to the doctor. As far as children are concerned, appearance is important, but in addition the pharmacist can ask the parent whether the child is generally 'well'. A child who is cheerful and energetic is unlikely to have anything other than a minor problem, whereas one who is quiet and listless, or who is fractious, irritable and feverish, might require referral.

The age of the patient is important because the pharmacist will consider some symptoms as potentially more serious according to age. For example, acute diarrhoea in an otherwise healthy adult could reasonably be treated by the pharmacist. However, such symptoms in a baby could produce dehydration more quickly; elderly patients are also at a higher risk of becoming dehydrated. Oral thrush is common in babies, less common in older children and adults; the pharmacist's decision about whether to treat or refer could therefore be influenced by age.

Age will play an important part in determining any treatment offered by the pharmacist. Some preparations are not recommended at all for use in children under 12 years of age, for example oral *ibuprofen* and *loperamide*. *Hydrocortisone* cream and ointment should not be recommended for children under 10 years old. Others must be given in a reduced dose or as a paediatric formulation and the pharmacist will thus consider recommendations carefully.

History

There are two aspects to the term 'history' in relation to responding to symptoms. First, the history of the symptom being presented and second, previous medical history. For example, does the patient have diabetes, hypertension or asthma? Patient medication records should be used to record relevant existing conditions.

Questioning about the history of a condition may be useful; how and when the problem began, how it has progressed and so on. If the patient has had the problem before, previous episodes should be asked about to determine the action taken by the patient and its degree of success. In recurrent mouth ulcers, for example, do the current ulcers resemble the previous ones, was the doctor or dentist seen on previous occasions, was any treatment prescribed or OTC medicine purchased and, if so, did it work?

In asking about the history, the timing of particular symptoms can give valuable clues as to possible causes. The attacks of heartburn which occur after going to bed or on stooping or bending down are indeed likely to be due to reflux, whereas those which happen during exertion such as exercise or heavy work may not be.

History-taking is particularly important when assessing skin disease. Pharmacists often think, erroneously, that recognition of the appearance of skin conditions is the most important factor in responding to such symptoms. In fact, many dermatologist would argue that history-taking is more important because some skin conditions resemble each other in appearance. Furthermore, the appearance may be altered during the course of the condition. For example, the use of a topical corticosteroid inappropriately on infected or infested skin may substantially change the appearance; allergy to ingredients such as local anaesthetics may produce a problem in addition to the original complaint. The pharmacist must know, therefore, which creams, ointments or lotions have been applied.

Other symptoms

Patients generally tend to complain about the symptoms which concern them most. The pharmacist should always ask whether the patient has noticed any other symptoms, or anything different from usual, because, for various reasons, patients may not volunteer all the important information. Embarrassment may be one such reason, so that patients experiencing rectal bleeding may only mention that they have piles or are constipated.

The importance or significance of symptoms may not be recognized by patients; for example, those who have constipation as a side effect from a tricyclic antidepressant will probably not mention their dry mouth because they can see no link or connection between the two problems.

Danger symptoms

These are the symptoms or combinations of symptoms which should ring warning bells for pharmacists because immediate referral to the doctor is required. Blood in the sputum, vomit, urine or faeces would be examples of such symptoms, as would unexplained weight loss. Danger symptoms are included and discussed in each section of this book so that their significance can be understood by the pharmacist.

Decision-making: Is referral required?

As a general rule, the following should make the pharmacist consider referring the patient to the doctor:

long duration of symptoms

recurring or worsening problems

severe pain

failed medication (one or more appropriate medicines used already, without improvement)

suspected adverse drug reactions (to prescription or OTC medicine)

danger symptoms.

For relevant sections of this book, the duration of symptoms beyond which the pharmacist should consider immediate referral is defined in the section *When to refer*. In addition, for relevant sections a *Treatment timescale* is included; this is the length of time for which the problem might be treated before the patient sees the doctor.

Some community pharmacists now use referral forms as an additional means of conveying information to the doctor with the patient. Several Health Authorities have introduced such forms and the National Pharmaceutical Association also supplies them. Discussions with local family doctors can assist the development of protocols and guidelines for referral and we recommend that pharmacists take the opportunity to develop such guidelines with their medical colleagues. Joint discussions of this sort can lead to effective two-way referral systems and local agreements about preferred treatments.

Treatment

The pharmacist's background in pharmacology, therapeutics and pharmaceutics gives a sound base on which to make logical treatment choices based on the individual patient's need, together with the characteristics of the medicine concerned. In addition to the effectiveness of the active ingredients included in the product, the pharmacist will need to consider potential interactions, cautions, contra-indications and adverse reaction profile of each constituent. With the increasing move to evidence-based practice, pharmacists need to think carefully about the effectiveness of the treatments they recommend. The situation with OTC medicines is complex in that patient preference plays a key part in the choice of preparation. However health professionals are under increasing pressure to justify their decisions and provide value for money. Some pharmacists have developed their own OTC formularies with preferred treatments which are recommended by pharmacists and their staff. In some areas these have been discussed with local GPs and practice nurses to cover the referral of patients from the GP practice to the pharmacy.

Patient medication records can play an important part in supporting the process of responding to symptoms. Research shows that only one in four pharmacists currently records OTC treatment on their PMR system. Yet such recording can complete the profile of medication and review of concurrent drug therapy can identify potential drug interactions and adverse effects.

Key interactions between OTC treatments and other drugs are included in each section of this book. The *British National Formulary* provides an alphabetical listing of drugs and interactions, together with an indication of clinical significance. In this book, generic drug names are italicized.

For symptoms discussed in this book, the section on *Management* includes brief information about the efficacy, advantages and disadvantages of possible therapeutic options. Also included are useful points of information for patients about the optimum use of OTC treatments, under the heading *Practical points*. In the case of antacids, for example, liquid preparations have a smaller particle size and cover a larger surface area more quickly than do tablets. From the point of view of convenience, however, the patient may prefer to have an antacid in both forms, the liquid to be taken at home and the tablets to carry around at work or while out of the house. Patients can also be advised of the best time to take an antacid preparation: dosing about 1 hour after meals will ensure that excess acid is neutralized and that the antacid will have a longer duration of action. Because the speed of stomach emptying will have decreased, the antacid will stay in the stomach and exert its effect for longer.

Outcome

Most of the symptoms dealt with by community pharmacist will be of a minor and self-limiting nature and should resolve within a few days.

However, sometimes this will not be the case and it is the pharmacist's responsibility to make sure that patients know what to do if they do not get better. Here, a defined timescale should be used, as suggested in relevant sections of this book, so that when offering treatment the pharmacist can set a time beyond which the patient should seek medical advice if symptoms do not improve. The *Treatment timescales* outlined in this book naturally vary according to the symptom and sometimes according to the patient's age, but are usually less than a week.

Privacy in the pharmacy

Roughly half of pharmacy customers feel that there is insufficient privacy in the shop to discuss personal matters. The pharmacist should always bear the question of privacy in mind and, where possible, seek to create an atmosphere of confidentiality if sensitive problems are to be discussed. Using professional judgement and personal experience, the pharmacist will quickly sense any embarrassment on the patient's part and can suggest moving to a quieter part of the premises to continue the conversation. The provision of a counselling area, where possible, may encourage embarrassed patients to seek advice more readily. Some Health Authorities are experimenting with premises investment schemes for community pharmacies and providing financial support for the installation of counselling areas and the necessary refitting or building.

Working with family doctors

Community pharmacists are the key gateway into the formal National Health Service (NHS) through their filtering of symptoms, with referral to the family doctor when necessary. Some community pharmacists are now working more closely with local GP practices by advising on prescribing. There is a great deal of scope for joint working in the area of OTC medicines. We suggest that pharmacists might consider the following steps.

Agreeing guidelines for referral with local family doctors, perhaps including feedback from the GP to the pharmacist on the outcome of the referral.

Using PMRs to keep information on OTC recommendations to patients.

Keeping local family doctors informed about prescription only medicine (POM) to pharmacy medicines (P) changes.

Using referral forms when recommending that a patient sees his or her doctor.

Agreeing an OTC formulary with local GPs and practice nurses.

Agreeing with local GPs the response to suspected adverse drug reactions.

Actions like these will help to improve communication, will increase the GP's confidence in the contribution the pharmacist can make to patient care and will also support the pharmacist's integration into the primary care team.

Respiratory Problems

Colds and flu

The common cold comprises a mixture of upper respiratory tract viral infections. Although colds are self-limiting many people choose to buy over-the-counter (OTC) medicines for symptomatic relief. Some of the ingredients of OTC cold remedies may interact with prescribed therapy, occasionally with serious consequences. Therefore, careful attention needs to be given to taking a medication history and selecting an appropriate product.

What you need to know
Age (approx)
Child or adult
Duration of symptoms
What are the symptoms
Runny/blocked nose
'Summer cold'
Sneezing/coughing
Generalized aches/headache
High temperature
Sore throat
Earache
Facial pain/frontal headache
Flu
Asthma
Previous history
Allergic rhinitis
Bronchitis
Heart disease
Present medication

Significance of questions and answers

Age

Establishing who the patient is, child or adult, is important. This will influence the pharmacist's decision about the necessity of referral to the doctor and choice of treatment. Children are more susceptible to upper respiratory tract infection than adults.

Duration

Patients may describe a rapid onset of symptoms or a gradual onset over several hours; the former is said to be more commonly true of flu, the latter of the common cold. Such guidelines are general rather than definitive. The symptoms of the common cold usually last for about 7 days. Some symptoms, such as a cough, may persist after the worst of the cold is over.

Symptoms

Runny/blocked nose

Most patients will experience a runny nose (rhinorrhoea). This is initially a clear watery fluid which is then followed by the production of thicker and more tenacious mucus (this may be purulent). Nasal congestion occurs because of dilation of blood vessels, leading to swelling of the lining surfaces of the nose. This narrows the nasal passages which are further blocked by increased mucus production.

'Summer colds'

These are where the main symptoms are nasal congestion, sneezing and irritant watery eyes and are more likely to be due to allergic rhinitis (see p. 42).

Sneezing/coughing

Sneezing occurs because the nasal passages are irritated and congested. A cough may be present (see p. 23) either because the pharynx is irritated (producing a dry, tickly cough) or as a result of irritation of the bronchus caused by post-nasal drip.

Aches and pains/headache

Headaches may be experienced because of inflammation and congestion of the nasal passages and sinuses. A persistent or worsening frontal headache (pain above or below the eyes) may be due to sinusitis (see below and p. 181). People with flu often report muscular and joint aches—this is more likely to occur with flu than the common cold (see below).

High temperature

Those suffering from a cold often complain of feeling hot, but in general a high temperature will not be present. The presence of fever may be an indication that the patient has flu rather than a cold (see below).

Sore throat

The throat often feels dry and sore during a cold and may sometimes be the first sign that a cold is imminent (see p. 34).

Earache

Earache is a common complication of colds, especially in children. When nasal catarrh is present the ear can feel blocked. This is due to blockage of the Eustachian tube, which is the tube connecting the middle ear to the back of the nasal cavity. Under normal circumstances the middle ear is an air-containing compartment. However, if the Eustachian tube is blocked the ear can no longer be 'cleared' by swallowing and may feel uncomfortable and deaf. This situation often resolves spontaneously, but decongestants and inhalations can be helpful (see *Management* below). Sometimes the situation worsens when the middle ear fills up with fluid. This is an ideal site for a secondary infection to settle. When this does occur the ear becomes acutely painful and usually requires antibiotics. The infection is called otitis media.

In summary, a blocked uncomfortable ear is often present and does not need referral providing it does not persist. A very painful ear needs referral.

Facial pain/frontal headache

This may signify sinusitis. Sinuses are air-containing spaces in the bony structures adjacent to the nose (maxillary sinuses) and above the eyes (frontal sinuses). In a cold their lining surfaces become inflamed and swollen, producing catarrh. The secretions drain into the nasal cavity. If the drainage passage becomes blocked, fluid builds up in the sinus and can become secondarily (bacterially) infected. If this happens, persistent pain arises in the sinus areas. The maxillary sinuses are most commonly involved. When the frontal sinuses are infected the sufferer may complain of a frontal (forehead) headache. The headache is typically worsened by lying down or bending forwards.

Flu

Flu often starts abruptly with hot and cold shivery feelings, muscular aches and pains in the limbs, a dry sore throat, cough and high temperature. These symptoms usually resolve over 3–5 days. There is often a period of generalized weakness and malaise following the worst of the symptoms. A dry cough may persist for some time.

Warning that complications are developing may be given by a severe or productive cough, persisting high fever, pleuritic-type chest pain (see p. 52) or delirium.

True influenza is relatively uncommon compared to the large number of flu-like infections that occur. Influenza is generally more unpleasant, although both usually settle with no need for referral.

Flu can be complicated by secondary lung infection (pneumonia). Complications are much more likely to occur in the very young, the very old and those who have pre-existing heart or lung disease (chronic bronchitis)

Asthma

Many asthmatic attacks can be triggered by such viral infections. Most asthma sufferers learn to start or increase their usual medication to prevent such an occurrence. However, if these measures fail then referral is recommended.

Previous history

Chronic bronchitis may be advised to see their doctor if they have a bad cold or flu-like infection as it is often complicated by a secondary chest infection. Also, many asthmatic attacks are triggered by upper respiratory tract viral infections. Certain medications are best avoided in those with heart disease, hypertension and diabetes.

Present medication

The pharmacist must ascertain any medicines being taken by the patient. It is important to remember that interactions might occur with some of the constituents of commonly used OTC medicines.

If medication has already been tried for relief of cold symptoms with no improvement and if the remedies tried were appropriate, referral to the doctor may be considered. In most cases of colds and flu OTC treatment will be appropriate.

When to refer
Earache
Facial pain/frontal headache
Flu
In the very young
In the very old
In those with heart or lung disease, e.g. chronic bronchitis
With persisting fever and productive cough
With delirium
With pleuritic chest pain; for further discussion see p. 52
Asthma

Treatment timescale

Once the pharmacist has recommended treatment, patients should be advised to see their doctor in a week if the cold has not improved.

Management

The use of OTC medicines in the treament of colds and flu is widespread and such products are heavily advertised to the public. There is little doubt that appropriate symptomatic treatment can make the patient feel better; the placebo effect also plays an important part here. The pharmacist's role is to select appropriate treatment based on the patient's symptoms. Polypharmacy abounds in the area of cold treatments and patients should not be 'over treated'. The discussion of medicines which follows is based on individual constituents; the pharmacist can decide whether a combination of two or more drugs is needed.

Decongestants

Sympathomimetics

Sympathomimetics (e.g. *pseudoephedrine* or *phenylpropanolamine*) can be effective in reducing nasal congestion. Nasal decongestants work by constricting the dilated blood vessels in the nasal mucosa. The nasal membranes are effectively shrunk, so that drainage of mucus and circulation of air are improved and the feeling of nasal stuffiness is relieved. These medicines can be given orally or applied topically. Tablets and syrups are available, as are nasal sprays and drops. If nasal sprays/drops are to be recommended, the pharmacist should advise the patient not to use the product for longer than 7 days. Rebound congestion (rhinitis medicamentosa) can occur with topically applied but not oral sympathomimetics. The decongestant effects of topical products containing *oxymetazoline* or *xylometazoline* are longer lasting (up to 6 hours) than those of some other preparations such as *ephedrine*. The pharmacist can give useful advice about the correct way to administer nasal drops and sprays.

Problems

The pharmacist should be aware that some of these drugs (e.g. *ephedrine, pseudoephedrine*) when taken orally have the potential to keep patients awake, because of their stimulating effects on the central nervous system (CNS). In general, *ephedrine* is more likely to produce this effect than the other sympathomimetics. It is reasonable to suggest that the patient avoids taking a dose of the medicine near bedtime.

Sympathomimetics can cause stimulation of the heart, an increase in blood pressure, and may affect diabetic control because they can increase blood glucose levels. They should not be used by diabetic patients, those with heart disease or hypertension, or those with hyperthyroidism. Hyperthyroid patients' hearts are more vulnerable to irregularity, so that stimulation of the heart is particularly undesirable for such patients.

Sympathomimetics are most likely to cause these unwanted effects when taken by mouth and are unlikely to do so when used topically. Nasal drops and sprays containing sympathomimetics can therefore be recommended for those patients in whom the oral drugs are to be avoided. Saline nasal drops or the use of inhalations would be other possible choices for patients in this group.

The interaction between sympathomimetics and monoamine oxidase inhibitors (MAOIs) is potentially extremely serious; a hypertensive crisis can be induced and several deaths have occurred in such cases. This interaction can occur up to 2 weeks after a patient has stopped taking the MAOI, so the pharmacist must established any recently discontinued medication.

There is a possibility that topically applied sympathomimetics could induce such a reaction in a patient taking an MAOI. It is therefore advisable to avoid both oral and topical sympathomimetics in patients taking MAOIs.

Contra-indications—avoid in those with:
   diabetes
   heart disease
   hypertension
   hyperthyroidism
Interactions—avoid in those taking:
   MAOIs (e.g. *phenelzine*)
   reversible inhibitors of monoamine oxidase A (RIMAs) (e.g.
      moclobemide)
   beta blockers
   guanethidine, *debrisoquine* or *bethanidine*
   tricyclic atidepressants (e.g. *amitriptyline*): a theoretical
      interaction which appears not to be a problem in practice.

Antihistamines (see also p. 46)

Antihistamines can reduce some of the symptoms of a cold; runny nose (rhinorrhoea) and sneezing. These effects are due to the anticholinergic action of antihistamines. The older drugs (e.g. *chlorpheniramine*, *promethazine*) have more pronounced anticholinergic actions than do the non-sedating antihistamines (e.g. *astemizole*, *terfenadine*, *loratadine*, *cetirizine*). Antihistamines are not so effective at reducing nasal congestion. Some (e.g. *diphenhydramine*) may also be included in cold remedies for their supposed antitussive action (see p. 29).

Interactions

The problem of using antihistamines, particularly the older types (e.g. *chlorpheniramine*), is that they can cause drowsiness. Alcohol will increase this effect, as will drugs which have the ability to cause drowsiness or CNS depression such as benzodiazepines, phenothiazines or barbiturates. Antihistamines with known sedative effects should never be recommended for anyone who is driving, or in whom an impaired level of consciousness may be dangerous (e.g. operators of machinery at work).

Because of their anticholinergic activity, the older antihistamines may produce the same adverse effects as anticholinergic drugs (i.e. dry mouth, blurred vision, constipation and urinary retention). These effects are more likely if antihistamines are given concurrently with anticholinergics such as *hyoscine*, or with drugs which have anticholinergic actions such as tricyclic antidepressants.

Antihistamines should be avoided in patients with prostatic hyper-trophy and closed-angle glaucoma because of possible anticholinergic side effects. Patients with closed-angle glaucoma should avoid anti-histamines because they may cause increased intra-ocular pressure.

Anti-cholinergic drugs can occasionally precipitate acute urinary retention in predisposed patients, for example men with prostatic hypertrophy.

While the probability of such serious adverse effects is low, the pharmacist should be aware of the origin of possible adverse effects from OTC medicines.

At high doses, antihistamines can produce stimulation rather than depression of the CNS. There have been occasional reports of fits being induced at very high doses of antihistamines and it is for this reason that it has been argued that they should be avoided in epileptic patients. However, this appears to be a theoretical rather than practical problem. In addition, *chlorpheniramine* has been reported to cause elevated serum *phenytoin* levels and there could be the risk of toxic effects when the two are given concurrently. Antihistamines can antagonize the effects of *betahistine*.

Interactions:
  alcohol
  hypnotics
  sedatives (including barbiturates)
  betahistine
  anticholinergics, e.g. *benzhexol*, tricyclics
  phenytoin

Side effects:
  drowsiness (driving, occupational hazard).
  constipation
  blurred vision.
Cautions:
  closed-angle glaucoma
  prostatic obstruction
  epilepsy
  liver disease.

Cough remedies
For discussion of products for the treatment of cough, see p. 27.

Analgesics
For details of analgesics, their uses and side effects, see p. 183.

Products for sore throats
For discussion of products for the treatment of sore throat, see p. 38.

Practical points

Diabetics
The National Pharmaceutical Association and the British Diabetic Association jointly publish a useful list of OTC products and their sugar and sweetener content. In short-term use for acute conditions, the sugar content of OTC medicines is less important.

Steam inhalations
These may be useful in reducing nasal congestion and soothing the air passages, particularly if a productive cough is present. For further discussion of their use, see p. 31. Inhalants which can be used on handkerchiefs, bedclothes and pillowcases are available. These usually contain aromatic ingredients such as *eucalyptus*. Such products can be useful in providing some relief but are not as effective as steam-based inhalations.

Nasal spray or drops?
Nasal sprays are preferable for adults and children aged over 6 years because the small droplets in the spray mist reach a large surface area. Drops are more easily swallowed, which increases the possibility of systemic effects.

For children aged under 6 years drops are to be preferred because in young children the nostrils are not sufficiently wide to allow the effective use of sprays. Paediatric versions of nasal drops should be used where appropriate. Manufacturers of paediatric drops advise consultation with the doctor for children under 2 years of age.

Colds and flu in practice

Case 1

A woman in her mid fifties asks what you can recommend for her husband. He has a very bad cold; the worst symptoms are his blocked nose and sore throat. Although his throat feels sore, she tells you there is only a slight reddening (she looked this morning). He has had the symptoms since last night and is not feverish. He does not have earache but has complained of a headache. When you ask her if he is taking any medicines she says yes, he is taking some tablets for his high blood pressure. They are pink, but she cannot remember what they are called. You check the patient medication record and find that he is taking propranolol 80 mg three times daily.

The pharmacist's view

This man has the symptoms of the common cold. They came on quickly and this woman's husband is concerned most with his congested nose and sore throat. He is taking antihypertensive medication so oral sympathomimetics are best avoided. You could recommend that he sucks a soothing lozenge or pastille for his sore throat and that he tries a topical decongestant or an inhalation to clear his blocked nose. She can be reassured that the symptoms will not last for more than a few days.

The doctor's view

The advice given by the pharmacist is sensible. A simple analgesic such as *paracetamol* could help the headache. The development of sinusitis at such an early stage in an infection would be unlikely but it would be wise to enquire whether his colds are usually uncomplicated and to ascertain the site of his headache.

Case 2

It is Saturday afternoon. A man in his twenties asks you to recommend some good ear drops for his little boy, Alan, aged 4 years. Alan had a cold a few days ago and is still complaining of earache, although all his other symptoms have gone. When you ask if the child otherwise seems well, Alan's father tells you that he looks flushed and seems hot and has been fractious and irritable for the last day or so. He and his wife are very worried about Alan.

The pharmacist's view

This is a 4-year-old child who is showing signs of an ear infection. In addition to his earache, the child seems generally unwell and may be feverish. Over-the-counter treatment is inappropriate in this case, except perhaps a recommendation of an analgesic/antipyretic until the child sees the doctor. *Paracetamol* could be given to Alan and his father should be advised to call the doctor if the symptoms worsen. Otherwise, Alan should be kept warm and comfortable, be given *paracetamol* regularly, and see the doctor on Monday.

The doctor's view

Ear drops are unlikely to be of any value as the story is suggestive of a middle ear infection (otitis media). If the symptoms do not settle with *paracetamol* it is likely that an antibiotic such as *amoxycillin* will need to be prescribed.

Cough

Coughing is a protective reflex action caused when the airway is being irritated or obstructed. Its purpose is to clear the airway so that breathing can continue normally. The majority of coughs presenting in the pharmacy will be caused by an upper respiratory viral infection. They will often be associated with other symptoms of a cold.

What you need to know

Age (approx)
  Baby, child, adult
Duration
Nature
  Dry or productive
Associated symptoms
  Cold, sore throat, fever
  Sputum production
  Chest pain
  Shortness of breath
  Wheeze
Previous history
  Chronic bronchitis
  Asthma
  Diabetes
  Heart disease
  Gastro-oesophageal reflux
Smoking habit
Present medication

Significance of questions and answers

Age
Establishing who is the patient, child or adult. This will influence the choice of treatment and whether referral is necessary.

Duration
Most coughs are self-limiting and will be better within a few days with or without treatment. In general, a cough of longer than 2 week's duration should be referred to the doctor for further investigation.

Nature of cough

Unproductive (dry, tickly or tight)

In an unproductive cough no sputum is produced. These coughs are usually caused by viral infection and are self-limiting.

Productive (chesty or loose)

Sputum is, of course, normally produced. It is an over-secretion of sputum which leads to coughing. Over-secretion may be caused by irritation of the airways due to infection, allergy, etc., or when the cilia are not working properly (e.g. in smokers). Non-coloured (clear or whitish) sputum is uninfected and known as 'mucoid'. Coloured sputum may indicate a chest infection such as bronchitis or pneumonia and require referral. In these situations the sputum is described as green, yellow or rusty-coloured thick mucus. Sometimes blood may be present in the sputum (haemoptysis), giving a colour ranging from pink to deep red. Blood may be an indication of a relatively minor problem such as a burst capillary following a bout of violent coughing during an acute infection but may be a warning of more serious problems. Haemoptysis is an indication for referral.

In heart failure and mitral stenosis the sputum is sometimes described as 'pink and frothy' or can be bright red. Confirming symptoms would be breathlessness (especially in bed during the night) and swollen ankles.

Tuberculosis (TB)

Until recently thought of as a disease of the past, the number of cases of TB has been increasing in the UK and there is increasing concern about resistant strains. Chronic cough with haemoptysis associated with chronic fever and night sweats are classical symptoms. TB is largely a disease of poverty and more likely to present in deprived communities.

Croup

This usually occurs in infants. The cough has a harsh barking quality. It develops a day or so after the onset of cold-like symptoms. It is often associated with difficulty with breathing and an inspiratory stridor (noise in throat on breathing in). Referral is necessary.

Whooping cough

This starts with catarrhal symptoms. The characteristic whoop is not present in the early stages of infection. The whoop is the sound produced when breathing in after a paroxysm of coughing. The bouts of coughing prevent normal breathing and the whoop represents the desperate attempt to get a breath in. Referral is necessary.

Associated symptoms

A cold, sore throat and catarrh may be associated with a cough. Often there may be a temperature and generalized muscular aches present. This would be in keeping with a viral infection and be self-limiting. Chest pain, shortness of breath or wheezing are all indications for referral (see p. 52).

Post-nasal drip

Post-nasal drip is a common cause of coughing and may be due to sinusitis (see p. 15).

Previous history

Certain cough remedies are best avoided in diabetics and anyone with heart disease or hypertension (see p. 30).

Chronic bronchitis

Questioning may reveal a history of chronic bronchitis which is being treated by the doctor with antibiotics. In this situation further treatment may be possible with an appropriate cough medicine.

Asthma

A recurrent night-time cough can indicate asthma, especially in children, and should be referred. Asthma may sometimes present as a chronic cough without wheezing. A family history of eczema, hay fever and asthma is worth asking about. Patients with such a family history appear to be more prone to extended episodes of coughing following a simple upper respiratory tract infection.

Cardiovascular

Coughing can be a symptom of heart failure (see p. 24). If there is a history of heart disease, especially with a persisting cough, then referral is advisable.

Gastro-oesophageal

Gastro-oesaphogeal reflux can cause coughing. Sometimes such reflux is asymptomatic apart from coughing.

Smoking habit

Smoking will exacerbate a cough and can cause coughing since it is irritant to the lungs. One in three long-term smokers develop a chronic cough. If coughing is recurrent and persistent the pharmacist is in a good position to offer health education advice about the benefits of stopping smoking, suggesting nicotine replacement therapy where appropriate. However, on stopping, the cough may initially become worse as the cleaning action of the cilia is re-established during the first few days and it is worth mentioning this. Smokers may assume their cough is harmless and it is always important to ask about any change in the nature of the cough which might suggest a serious cause.

Present medication

It is always essential to establish which medicines are currently being taken. This includes those prescribed by a doctor and any bought over the counter (OTC), 'borrowed' from a friend or neighbour or 'rediscovered' in the family medicine chest. It is important to remember the possibility of interactions with cough medicine.

It is also useful to know which cough medicines have been tried already. The pharmacist may decide that an inappropriate preparation has been taken, for example a cough suppressant for a productive cough. If one or more appropriate remedies have been tried without success then referral is advisable.

Angiotensin-converting enzyme (ACE) inhibitors

Chronic coughing may occur in patients, particularly women, taking ACE inhibitors such as *enalapril, captopril* and *lisinopril*. The problem is now well recognized and patients may develop the cough within days of starting treatment or after a period of a few weeks or even months. The exact incidence of the reaction is not known and estimates vary from 2 to 10% of patients taking ACE inhibitors. Typically the cough is irritating, non-productive and persistent. Any ACE inhibitor may induce coughing and there seems to be little advantage to be gained in changing from one to another. The cough may resolve or may persist; in some patients the cough is so troublesome and distressing that ACE inhibitor therapy may have to be discontinued. Any patients in whom medication is suspected as the cause of a cough should be referred to their doctor.

When to refer	
Cough lasting 2 weeks or more	
Sputum (yellow, green, rusty or blood-stained)	
Chest pain	
Shortness of breath	
Wheezing	For further details,
Whooping cough or croup	see p. 52
Recurrent nocturnal cough	
Suspected adverse drug reaction	
Failed medication	

After a series of questions the pharmacist should be in a position to decide whether treatment or referral is the best option.

Treatment timescale

Once the pharmacist has recommended an appropriate treatment patients should see their doctor after 5 days if the cough has not improved.

Management

Pharmacists are well aware of the debate about the clinical efficacy of the cough remedies available OTC. In particular, the lack of scientific evidence that expectorants have any effect and the use of combinations with apparently contradictory ingredients have been cited.

However, many people who visit the pharmacy for advice do so because they want some relief from their symptoms and, while the effectiveness of cough remedies remains unproven, there is no doubt that they at least have a valuable placebo effect.

The choice of treatment depends on the type of cough. Suppressants (e.g. *pholcodine*) are effective in treating unproductive coughs, while expectorants such as *guaiphenesin* in theory should be effective in the treatment of productive coughs. The pharmacist should check that the preparation contains an appropriate dose, since some products contain sub-therapeutic amounts. Demulcents like *simple linctus,* which soothe the throat, are particularly useful in children and pregnant women as they contain no active ingredients.

Productive coughs should not be treated with cough suppressants because the result is pooling and retention of mucus in the lungs and a higher chance of infection, especially in chronic bronchitis.

There is no logic in using expectorants (which promote coughing) and suppressants (which reduce coughing) together—they have opposing effects. Therefore, products which contain both are not therapeutically sound.

Cough suppressants

Codeine/pholcodine

Both are effective cough suppressants. *Pholcodine* has several advantages over *codeine* in that it produces fewer side effects (even at OTC doses *codeine* can cause constipation and, at high doses, respiratory depression) and *pholcodine* is less liable to abuse. For these reasons, *codeine* is best avoided in the treatment of children's coughs and should never be used in children under a year old. Both *pholcodine* and *codeine* can induce drowsiness, although in practice this does not appear to be a problem. Nevertheless it is sensible to give an appropriate warning. *Codeine* is well known as a drug of abuse and many pharmacists choose not to recommend it. Sales often have to be refused because of knowledge or likelihood of abuse. *Pholcodine* can be given at a dose of 5 mg to children aged over 2 years (5 mg of *pholcodine* is contained in 5 ml of *pholcodine linctus B.P.*). Adults may take doses of up to 15 mg up to three or four times daily. The drug has a long half-life and may be more appropriately given as a twice-daily dose.

Dextromethorphan

This is a less potent cough suppressant than *pholcodine* and *codeine* but is effective. It is generally non-sedating and has few side effects. Occasionally drowsiness had been reported but, as for *pholcodine*, this does not seem to be a problem in practice. *Dextromethorphan* can be given to children of 2 years old and over. *Dextrometharphan* was generally thought to have a low potential for abuse. However, there have been rare reports of mania following abuse and consumption of very large quantities and pharmacists should be aware of this possibility if regular purchases are made.

Demulcents

Preparations such as *glycerin, lemon and honey* or *simpe linctus* are popular remedies and are useful for their soothing effect. They do not contain any active ingredient and are considered to be safe in children and pregnant women. Their pleasant taste makes them particularly suitable for children but their high syrup content should be noted.

Expectorants

Two mechanisms have been proposed for expectorants. They may act directly by stimulating bronchial mucus secretion, leading to increased liquefying of sputum, making it easier to cough up. Alternatively, they may act indirectly via irritation of the gastrointestinal (GI) tract which has a subsequent action on the respiratory system resulting in increased mucus secretion. This latter theory has less convincing evidence than the former to support it.

Guiphenesin

This is commonly found in cough remedies. In adults, the dose required to produce expectoration is 100–200 mg, so in order to have a theoretical chance of effectiveness any product recommended should contain a sufficiently high dose. Some OTC preparations contain sub-therapeutic doses. In the USA, the Food and Drugs Administration (FDA, the licensing body) reviewed OTC medicines and evidence from studies supporting *guaiphenesin* was sufficiently strong enough for the FDA to be convinced of its efficacy.

Ipecacuanha

This has been used as an expectorant for many years and is found in several formulary preparations. Such preparations have now fallen out of favour and the only one with a logical formulation is *ammonia and ipecacuanha mixture (mist. expect.)* where the other constituent *(ammonium bicarbonate)* is also said to have an expectorant action.

Ammonium salts

Ammonium chloride and *ammonium bicarbonate* were traditionally used as expectorants in formulary mixtures such as *ammonia and ipecacuanha mixture*. The only such preparations prescribable on the National Health Service (NHS) in the UK are *ammonia and ipecacuanha mixture* and *ammonium chloride mixture*. The latter's intended use was originally acidification of urine. Problems which can ensue from the use of *ammonium chloride mixture* include vomiting and acidosis. The mixture also has an extremely unpleasant taste. From the pharmacist's point of view, there are other expectorant mixtures which are more acceptable to patients and less liable to cause side effects.

Cough remedies: Other constituents

Antihistamines

Examples used in OTC products include *diphenhydramine* and *promethazine*. Theoretically these reduce the frequency of coughing and have a drying effect on secretions, but in practice they also induce drowsiness. Combinations of antihistamines with expectorants are illogical and best avoided. A combination of an antihistamine and a cough suppressant may be useful in that antihistamines can help to dry up secretions and, when the combination is given as a night-time dose if the cough is disturbing sleep, a good night's sleep will invariably follow. This is one of the rare occasions when a side effect proves useful. The non-sedating antihistamines are less effective in symptomatic treatment of coughs and colds because of their less pronounced anticholinergic actions.

Interactions. Traditional antihistamines should not be taken by patients who are taking phenothiazines and tricyclic antidepressants because of additive anticholinergic and sedative effects. Increased sedation will also occur with barbiturates (e.g. where these are used in epileptic therapy) or any other drug which has a central nervous system (CNS) depressant effect. Alcohol should be avoided because this will also lead to increased drowsiness. See p. 47 for more details of interactions, side effects and contra-indications of antihistamines.

Interactions:
  alcohol
  hypnotics/anxiolytics
  sedatives.
Side effects:
  drowsiness.
Cautions:
  closed-angled glaucoma, prostatic hypertrophy.

Sympathomimetics

Examples include *pseudoephedrine* and *phenylpropanolamine*. These are commonly included in cough and cold remedies (see also p. 17) for their bronchodilatory and decongestant actions. *Phenylpropanolamine* is a weaker bronchodilator than *ephedrine* and *pseudoephedrine*. All three have a stimulant effect which may lead to a sleepless night if taken close to bedtime. They may be useful if the patient has a blocked nose as well as a cough and an expectorant/decongestant combination can be useful in productive coughs. These drugs can cause raised blood pressure, stimulation of the heart and alterations in diabetic control.

Oral sympathomimetics should not be recommended for patients with:
  diabetes
  coronary heart disease (e.g. angina)
  hypertension
  hyperthyroidism.
Interactions—sympathomimetics should be avoided by patients taking:
  monoamine oxidase inhibitors (MAOIs) (e.g. *phenelzine)*
  reversible inhibitors of monoamineoxidase A (RIMAs) (e.g.
    moclobemide)
  beta blockers
  guanethidine, debrisoquine or *bethanidine*
  tricylic antidepressants (e.g. *amitriptyline*); a theoretical interaction
    which does not seem to cause problems in practice.

Theophylline

This is sometimes included in cough remedies for its bronchodilator effect. Over-the-counter medicines containing *theophylline* should not be taken at the same time as prescribed theophylline since toxic blood levels and side effects may occur. The action of *theophylline* can be potentiated by some drugs, for example *cimetidine* and *erythromycin*.

Now that *cimetidine* can be purchased OTC, remember to check other OTC medicines being taken.

Levels of *theophylline* in the blood are reduced by smoking and drugs such as *carbamazepine, phenytoin* and *rifampicin* which induce liver enzymes, so that the metabolism of *theophylline* is increased and lower serum levels result.

Side effects include gastrointestinal (GI) irritation, nausea, palpitations, insomnia and headaches. The adult dose is typically 120 mg three or four times daily. It is not recommended in children. Before selling any OTC product containing *theophylline,* check that the patient is not already taking the drug on prescription. If the patient is, do not recommend a product containing *theophylline.*

Practical points

Diabetics

Current thinking is that in short-term acute conditions the amount of sugar in cough medicines is relatively unimportant. Diabetic control is often upset during infections and the additional sugar is not now considered to be a major problem. Nevertheless many diabetic patients may prefer a sugar-free product, as will many other customers who wish to reduce sugar intake for themselves and their children, and many such products are now available. As part of their contribution to improving dental health, pharmacists can ensure that they stock and display a range of sugar-free medicines.

Steam inhalations

These can be very useful, particularly in productive coughs. The steam helps to liquefy lung secretions and patients find the warm moist air comforting. While there is no evidence that the addition of medications to the water produces a better clinical effect than steam alone, some may prefer to add a preparation such as *Friar's balsam* or *menthol and eucalyptus* or a proprietary inhalant. One teaspoonful of inhalant should be added to a pint of hot (not boiling) water and the steam inhaled. Apart from the risk from scalding, boiling water volatilizes the constituents too quickly. A cloth or towel can be put over the head to trap the steam.

Fluid intake

Maintaining a high fluid intake helps to hydrate the lungs and hot drinks can have a soothing effect. General advice to patients with coughs and colds should be to increase fluid intake by around 2 litres a day.

Coughs in practice

Case 1

A woman aged about 30 asks what you can recommend for a cough. On questioning you find out that her son Steven, aged 6, has had a cough for 2 weeks. He gets it at night and it is disturbing his sleep although he doesn't seem to be troubled during the day. The cough is not productive and she has given Steven some *Buttercup Syrup* before he goes to bed but the cough is no better. Steven is not taking any other medicines. He has no pain on breathing nor shortness of breath. He has not had a cold recently but has had this kind of cough before.

The pharmacist's view

This is a 6-year-old child who has a night-time cough of 2 weeks' duration. Two facts suggest that referral to the doctor would be advisable. First, the cough is only present during the night, and second, Steven has had these symptoms before. A recurrent cough in a child at night can be a symptom of asthma, even if wheezing is not present. It is possible that the cough is occurring as a result of bronchial irritation following his recent viral upper respiratory tract infection. Such a cough can last for up to 6 weeks and is more likely to occur in those who have asthma or a family history of atopy (a predisposition to sensitivity to certain common allergens such as house dust mite, animal dander and pollen).

The doctor's view

Asthma is an obvious possibility. It would be interesting to know if anyone else in the family suffers from asthma, hay fever or eczema and whether Steven has ever had hay fever or eczema. Any of these features would make the diagnosis more likely. Mild asthma may present in this way without the usual symptoms of shortness of breath and wheezing.

An alternative diagnosis could still include an upper respiratory viral infection. Most coughs are more troublesome and certainly more obvious during the night. This can falsely give the impression that the cough is only nocturnal. It should also be remembered that both diagnoses can be correct, as a viral infection often initiates an asthmatic reaction. As there is uncertainty as to the diagnosis and specific bronchodilators may be appropriate, referral to the doctor is advisable.

If, after further history-taking and examination, the doctor feels that asthma is a possibility then treatment would be based on the British Thoracic Society guidelines, which are summarized in the *British National Formulary*. Naturally this would only be done after full discussion and agreement with the parents. Many parents are loath to have their child labelled as an asthma sufferer. The next problem is to prescribe a suitable inhalation device for a 6-year-old child. This may be an inhaler with a spacer device or a breath-actuated inhaler or a dry-powder inhaler. It would be usual to try a twice-daily dosage for 2–3 weeks and then review for future management.

Case 2

A man aged about 25 asks if you can recommend something for his cough. He sounds as if he has a bad cold and looks a bit pale. You find out that he has had the cough for a few days, with a blocked nose and a sore throat. He has no pain on breathing nor shortness of breath. The cough was chesty to begin with but he tells you it is now 'tickly and irritating'. He has not tried any medicines and is not taking any medicines from the doctor.

The pharmacist's view

This patient has the symptoms of the common cold and none of the danger signs associated with a cough that would make referral necessary. He is not taking any medicines, so the choice of possible treatments is wide. You could recommend something to treat his congested nose as well as his cough, for example, a cough suppressant and a sympatho-mimetic. *Pholcodine linctus* and a systemic or topical decongestant would be my choice. If I recommended a topical decongestant I would warn him to use it for no longer than a week to avoid the possibility of rebound congestion.

The doctor's view

The action suggested by the pharmacist is very reasonable. It may be worthwhile explaining that he is suffering from a viral infection which is self-limiting and should be better within a few days. If he is a smoker it would be an ideal time to encourage him to stop.

Sore throat

Most sore throats which present in the pharmacy will be caused by viral infection (90%), with only one in 10 being due to bacterial infection so that treatment with antibiotics is unnecessary in most cases. Clinically it is almost impossible to differentiate between the two. Most infections are self-limiting. Sore throats are often associated with other symptoms of a cold.

Once the pharmacist has excluded more serious conditions, an appropriate over-the-counter (OTC) medicine can be recommended.

What you need to know
Age (approx)
Baby, child, adult
Duration
Severity
Associated symptoms
Cold, congested nose, cough
Difficulty in swallowing
Hoarseness
Fever
Previous history
Smoking habit
Present medication

Significance of questions and answers

Age

Establishing who the patient is will influence the choice of treatment and whether referral is necessary. Streptococcal (bacterial) throat infections are more likely in children of school age.

Duration

Most sore throats are self-limiting and will be better within 7–10 days. If a sore throat has been present for longer, then the patient should be referred to the doctor for further advice.

Severity

If the sore throat is described as being extremely painful, especially in the absence of cold, cough and catarrhal symptoms, then referral should be recommended if there is no improvement within 24–48 hours.

Associated symptoms

A cold, catarrh and a cough may be associated with a sore throat. There may also be a fever and general aches and pains. These are in keeping with a minor self-limiting viral infection.

Hoarseness of longer than 3 weeks' duration and difficulty in swallowing (dysphagia) are both indications for referral.

Previous history

Recurrent bouts of infection (tonsillitis) would mean that referral is best. If the patient is diabetic, sugar-free medication might be preferred.

Smoking habit

Smoking will exacerbate a sore throat and if the patient smokes it can be a good time to offer advice and information about quitting. Remember that two-thirds of people who smoke want to stop.

Present medication

The pharmacist should establish whether any medication has been tried already to treat the symptoms. If one or more medicines have been tried without improvement, then referral to the doctor should be considered.

Current prescriptions are important and the pharmacist should question the patient carefully about them. Steroid inhalers (e.g. *beclomethasone* or *budesonide*) can cause hoarseness and candidal infections of the throat and mouth. Generally they tend to do this at high doses. Such infections can be prevented by rinsing the mouth with water after using the inhaler. It is also worthwhile checking the inhaler technique. Poor technique with metered-dose inhalers can lead to large amounts of the inhaled drug being deposited at the back of the throat. If you suspect this is the problem, discuss with the doctor whether a device which will help coordination or perhaps a different inhaler might be needed.

Any patient taking *carbimazole* and presenting with a sore throat should be referred immediately. A rare side effect of *carbimazole* is agranulocytosis (suppression of white cell production in the bone marrow). The same principle applies to any drug which can cause agranulocytosis. A sore throat in such patients can be the first sign of a life-threatening infection.

Symptoms for direct referral

Hoarseness

This is caused when there is inflammation of the vocal cords in the larynx (laryngitis). Laryngitis is typically caused by a self-limiting viral infection. It is usually associated with a sore throat and a hoarse, diminished voice. Antibiotics are of no value and symptomatic advice (see *Management* below), which includes resting the voice, should be given. The infection usually settles within a few days and referral is not necessary.

When this infection occurs in babies, infants or small children it can cause croup (acute laryngotracheitis) and present difficulty in breathing and stridor (see p. 24). In this situation referral is essential.

When hoarseness persists for more than 3 weeks, especially when it is not associated with an acute infection, referral is necessary. There are many causes of peristent hoarseness, some of which are serious. For example laryngeal cancer can present in this way and hoarseness may be the only early symptom. A doctor will normally refer the patient to an ear, nose and throat (ENT) specialist for accurate diagnosis.

Dysphagia

Difficulty in swallowing can occur in severe throat infection. It can happen when an abscess develops in the region of the tonsils (quinsy) as a complication of tonsillitis. This will usually result in a hospital admission where an operation to drain the abscess may be necessary and high-dose parenteral antibiotics may be given.

Glandular fever (infectious mononucleosis) is one viral cause of sore throat which often produces marked discomfort and may cause dysphagia. Referral is necessary for accurate diagnosis.

Most bad sore throats will cause discomfort on swallowing but not true difficulty and do not necessarily need referral unless there are other reasons for concern. Dysphagia when not associated with a sore throat always needs referral (see p. 67).

Appearance of throat

It is commonly thought that the presence of white spots, exudates or pus on the tonsils is an indication for referral or a means of differentiating between viral and bacterial infection, but this is not always so. Unfortunately the appearance can be the same in both types of infection and sometimes the throat can appear almost normal without exudates in a streptococcal (bacterial) infection.

Thrush

An exception not to be forgotten is candidal (thrush) infection which produces white plaques. However, these are rarely confined to the throat alone and are most commonly seen in babies or the very elderly. It is an unusual infection in younger adults and may be associated with more serious disorders which interfere with the body's immune system for example leukaemia, human immunodeficiency virus (HIV) and acquired immune deficiency syndrome (AIDS), or with immunosuppressive therapy (e.g. steroids). The plaques may be seen in the throat and on the gums and tongue. When they are scraped off the surface is raw and inflamed. Referral is advised if thrush is suspected and the throat is sore and painful. See p. 259 for more information about oral thrush.

Glandular fever

This is a viral throat infection caused by the Epstein–Barr virus. It is well known because of its tendency to leave its victims debilitated for some months afterwards and its association with the controversial condition myalgic encephalomyelitis (ME). The infection typically occurs in teenagers and young adults, with peak incidence between the ages of 14 and 21. It is known as the 'kissing disease'! A severe sore throat may follow a week or two of general malaise. The throat may become very inflamed with creamy exudates present. There may be difficulty in swallowing because of the painful throat. Glands (lymph nodes) in the neck and axillae (armpits) may be enlarged and tender. The diagnosis can be confirmed with a blood test, although this may not become positive until a week after the onset of the illness. Antibiotics are of no value; in fact if *ampicillin* is given during the infection a measles-type rash is likely to develop in 80% of those with glandular fever. Treatment is aimed at symptomatic relief.

When to refer
Sore throat lasting a week or more
Recurrent bouts of infection
Hoarseness of more than 3 weeks' duration
Difficulty in swallowing (dysphagia)
Failed medication

Treatment timescale

Patients should see their doctor in 5 days if the sore throat has not improved.

Management

Most sore throats are caused by viral infections and are self-limiting in nature. The pharmacist can offer a selection of treatments aimed at providing some relief from discomfort and pain until the infection subsides. Pastilles and lozenges to be sucked and mouthwashes or mouth sprays are the mainstays of treatment. Systemic analgesics may sometimes be useful (see p. 183 for discussion of available preparations).

Mouthwashes and sprays

Antiseptic (e.g. chlorhexidine)

A range of antiseptic mouthwashes is available OTC and research suggests that some preparations are more effective than others. Those containing *chlorhexidine, hexetidine, povidone-iodine* and *cetylpyridinium chloride* have been shown to have an effective antimicrobial action. Such preparations are unlikely to have antiviral activity, but would be useful where there was bacterial involvement. Mouthwashes and gargles are popular treatments and their placebo effect may also be useful.

Anti-inflammatory (e.g. benzydamine)

Benzydamine is an anti-inflammatory agent which is absorbed through the skin and mucosa and has been shown to be effective in reducing pain and inflammation in conditions of the mouth and throat. Side effects have occasionally been reported and include numbness and stinging of the mouth and throat. *Benzydamine* spray can be used in children of 6 years of age and over, whereas the mouthwash may only be recommended for children aged over 12.

Local anaesthetic (e.g. phenol, benzocaine)

Phenol has a local anaesthetic effect when applied to the mucosa and can be effective in reducing pain in sore throats. *Phenol*-based mouthwashes and sprays are available OTC. *Benzocaine* is available as a throat spray.

Lozenges and pastilles

These can be divided into three categories:
    antiseptic (e.g. *cetylpyridinium)*
    antifungal (e.g. *dequalinium)*
    local anaesthetic (e.g. *benzocaine).*

Lozenges and pastilles are commonly used OTC treatments for sore throats and, where viral infection is the cause, the main use of anti-bacterial and antifungal preparations is to soothe and moisten the throat.

Lozenges containing *cetylpyridinium cloride* have been shown to have an effective antibacterial action.

Local anaesthetic lozenges will numb the tongue and throat and can help to ease soreness and pain. *Benzocaine* can cause sensitization and such reactions have sometimes been reported.

Caution

Iodized throat lozenges should be avoided in pregnancy because they have the potential to affect the thyroid gland of the foetus.

Practical points

Diabetics

Mouthwashes and gargles are suitable and can be recommended. Sugar-free pastilles are available but the sugar content of such products is now not considered so important in short-term use.

Mouthwashes and gargles

Patients should be reminded that mouthwashes and gargles should not be swallowed. The potential toxicity of OTC products of this type is low and it is unlikely that problems would result from swallowing small amounts. However, there is a small risk of systemic toxicity from swallowing products containing iodine.

Manufacturers' recommendations about whether to use the mouthwash diluted or undiluted should be checked and appropriate advice given to the patient.

Analgesics

The pharmacist might recommend that the patient takes a simple analgesic such as paracetamol if the throat is very sore.

Sore throats in practice

Case 1

A woman comes to ask your advice about her son's very sore throat. He is 15 years old and is at home in bed. She says he has a temperature and that she can see creamy white matter at the back of his throat. He seems lethargic and hasn't been eating very well because his throat has been so painful. The sore throat started about 5 days ago and he has been in bed since yesterday. The glands on his neck are swollen and he has been complaining of pain in his abdomen.

The pharmacist's view

It would be best for this woman's son to be seen by the doctor. The symptoms appear to be severe and he is sufficiently ill enough to be in bed. Glandular fever is common in this age group and is a possibility. In the meantime you might consider recommending some *paracetamol* in soluble or syrup form to make it easier to swallow. The analgesic and antipyretic effects would both be useful in this case.

The doctor's view

The pharmacist is sensible in recommending referral. The description suggests a severe tonsillitis which will be caused by either a bacterial or viral infection. If it turns out to be viral, then glandular fever is a strong possibility. The doctor should check out the ideas, concerns and expectations of the mother and son and then explain the likely causes and treatment. Often it is not possible to rule out a bacterial (streptococcal) infection at this stage and it is safest to prescribe *oral penicillin,* or *erythromycin* if the patient is allergic to *penicillin.* Depending on the availability of laboratory services the doctor may take a throat swab which would identify a bacterial infection. If the infection has gone on for nearly a week then a blood test can identify infectious mononucleosis (glandular fever). Although there is no specific treatment for glandular fever, it is helpful for the patient to know what is going on and when to expect full recovery.

Case 2

A teenage girl comes into your shop with her mother. The girl has a sore throat which started yesterday. There is slight reddening of the throat. Her mother tells you she had a slight temperature during the night. She also has a blocked nose and has been feeling general 'aching'. She has no difficulty in swallowing and is not taking any medicines either prescribed or OTC.

The pharmacist's view

It sounds as though this girl has a minor upper respiratory tract infection. The symptoms described should remit within a few days. In the meantime, it would be reasonable to recommend some throat lozenges containing a local anaesthetic and to consider treatment for the other symptoms which are a blocked nose and generalized aching. A systemic analgesic would be helpful, perhaps in combination with a decongestant.

The doctor's view

The pharmacist's assessment sounds correct. Because she has a blocked nose, a viral infection is most likely. Many patients attend their doctor with similar symptoms hoping for a quick cure with antibiotics, which have no place in such infections.

Case 3

A middle-aged woman comes to ask your advice about her husband's bad throat. He has had a hoarse gruff voice for about a month and has tried various lozenges and pastilles without success. He has been a heavy smoker (at least a pack a day) for over 20 years and works as a bus driver.

The pharmacist's view

This woman should be advised that her husband should see his doctor. The symptoms which have been described are not those of a minor throat infection. On the basis of the long duration of the problem and of the unsuccessful use of several OTC treatments, it would be best for this man to see his doctor for further investigation.

The doctor's view

A persistent alteration in voice, gruff or hoarse, is an indication for referral to an ENT specialist. This man should have his vocal cords examined, which requires skill and special equipment that most family doctors do not have. It is possible he may have a cancer on his vocal cords (larynx), especially as he is a smoker.

Allergic rhinitis

Seasonal allergic rhinitis (hay fever) affects 10–15% of people in the UK and millions of patients rely on over-the-counter (OTC) medicines for treatment. The symptoms of allergic rhinitis occur after an inflammatory response involving the release of histamine which is initiated by allergens being deposited on the nasal mucosa. Allergens responsible for seasonal allergic rhinitis include grass pollens, tree pollens and fungal mould spores. Perennial allergic rhinitis occurs when symptoms are present all year round and is commonly caused by the house-dust mite, animal dander and feathers. Some patients may suffer from perennial rhinitis which becomes worse in the summer months.

What you need to know

Age (approx)
    Baby, child, adult
Duration
Symptoms
    Rhinorrhoea (runny nose)
    Nasal congestion
    Nasal itching
    Watery eyes
    Irritant eyes
    Discharge from the eyes
    Sneezing
Previous history
Associated conditions
    Eczema
    Asthma
Medication

Significance of questions and answers

Age

Symptoms of allergic rhinitis may start at any age, although its onset is more common in children and young adults (the condition is most common in those in their twenties and thirties). There is frequently a family history of atopy in allergic rhinitis sufferers. Thus children of allergic rhinitis sufferers are more likely to have the condition. The condition often improves or resolves as the child gets older. The age of the patient must be taken into account if any medication is to be recommended.

Young adults who may be taking examinations should be borne in mind, because treatment which may cause drowsiness is best avoided in these patients.

Duration

Sufferers will often present with seasonal rhinitis as soon as the pollen count becomes high. Symptoms may start in April when tree pollens appear and the hay fever season may start a month earlier in the south than in the north of England. Hay fever peaks between the months of May and July, when grass pollen levels are highest and spells of good weather commonly cause patients to seek the pharmacist's advice. Anyone presenting with a 'summer cold', perhaps of several weeks' duration, may be suffering from hay fever. Fungal spores are also a cause and are present slightly later, often until September.

People can suffer from what they think are mild cold symptoms for a long period, without knowing they have perennial rhinitis.

Symptoms

Rhinorrhoea

A runny nose is a commonly experienced symptom of allergic rhinitis. The discharge is often thin, clear and watery, but can change to a thicker, coloured, purulent one. This suggests a secondary infection, although the treatment for allergic rhinitis is not altered. There is no need for antibiotic treatment.

Nasal congestion

The inflammatory response caused by the allergen produces vasodilation of the nasal blood vessels and so results in nasal congestion. Severe congestion may result in headache and occasionally earache. Secondary infection such as otitis media and sinusitis can occur (see p. 15).

Nasal itching

This commonly occurs. Irritation is sometimes experienced on the roof of the mouth.

Eye symptoms

The eyes may be itchy and also watery; it is thought these symptoms are a result of tear duct congestion and also a direct effect of pollen grains being caught in the eye, setting off a local inflammatory response. Irritation of the nose by pollen probably contributes to eye symptoms too. People who suffer severe symptoms of allergic rhinitis may be hypersensitive to bright light (photophobic) and find that wearing dark glasses is helpful.

Sneezing

In hay fever the allergic response usually starts with symptoms of sneezing, then rhinorrhoea, progressing to nasal congestion. Classically, symptoms of hay fever are more severe in the morning and in the evening. This is because pollen rises during the day after being released in the morning and then settles at night. Patients may also describe a worsening of the condition on windy days as pollen is scattered and a reduction in symptoms when it rains, or after rain, as the pollen clears. Conversely, in those allergic to fungal mould spores the symptoms worsen in damp weather.

Previous history

There is commonly a history of hay fever going back over several years. However, it can occur at any age, so the absence of any previous history does not necessarily indicate that allergic rhinitis is not the problem. The incidence of hay fever has risen during the last decade. Pollution, particularly in urban areas, is thought to be at least partly responsible for the trend.

Perennial rhinitis can usually be distinguished from seasonal rhinitis by questioning about the timing and the occurrence of symptoms. People who have had hay fever before will often consult the pharmacist when symptoms are exacerbated in the summer months.

Danger symptoms/associated conditions

When associated symptoms such as tightness of the chest, wheezing, shortness of breath or coughing are present, then immediate referral is advised. These symptoms may herald the onset of an asthmatic attack.

Wheezing

Difficulty with breathing, possibly with a cough, suggests an asthmatic attack. Some suffers only experience asthma attacks during the hay fever season (seasonal asthma). These episodes can be quite severe and require referral. Seasonal asthmatics often do not have appropriate medication at hand as their attacks occur so infrequently, which puts them at greater risk.

Earache and facial pain

As with colds and flu (see p. 15) allergic rhinitis can be complicated by secondary bacterial infection in the middle ear (otitis media) or the sinuses (sinusitis). Both these conditions cause persisting severe pain.

Purulent conjunctivitis

Irritant watery eyes are a common accompaniment to allergic rhinitis. Occasionally this allergic conjuctivitis is complicated by a secondary infection. When this occurs the eyes become more painful (gritty sensation) and redder, and the discharge changes from being clear and watery to coloured and sticky (purulent). Referral is needed.

Medication

The pharmacist must establish whether any prescription or OTC medicines are being taken by the patient. Potential interactions between prescribed medication and antihistamines can therefore be identified.

It would be useful to know if any medicines have been tried already to treat the symptoms, especially where there is a previous history of allergic rhinitis. In particular, the pharmacist should be aware of the potentiation of drowsiness by some antihistamines combined with other medicines. This can lead to increased danger in certain occupations and driving.

Failed medication

If symptoms are not adequately controlled with OTC preparations then an appointment with the doctor may be worthwhile. Such an appointment is useful to explore the patient's beliefs and preconceptions about hay fever and its management. It is also an opportunity to suggest ideas for the next season.

When to refer
Wheezing and shortness of breath
Tightness of chest
Painful ear
Painful sinuses
Purulent conjunctivitis
Failed medication

Treatment timescale

Improvement in symptoms should occur within a few days. If no improvement is noted after 5 days, the patient might be referred to the doctor for other therapy.

Management

Management options include antihistamines, nasal steroids and *cromoglycate* in formulations for the nose and eyes. Over-the-counter antihistamines and steroid nasal sprays can be very effective in the treatment of allergic rhinitis. The choice of treatment should be rational and based on the patient's symptoms and previous history where relevant.

Many cases of hayfever can be managed with OTC treatment and it is reasonable for the pharmacist to recommend treatment. Patients with symptoms which do not respond to OTC products can be referred to the doctor at a later stage. Pharmacists also have an important role in ensuring that patients know how to use any prescribed medicines correctly (e.g. steroid nasal sprays, which must be used continuously for the patient to benefit).

Antihistamines

Most pharmacists would consider these drugs to be the first-line treatment for mild to moderate and intermittent symptoms of allergic rhinitis. They are effective in reducing sneezing and rhinorrhoea, less so in reducing nasal congestion. Non-sedating antihistamines available OTC include *astemizole, cetirizine and loratadine*. All are effective in reducing the troublesome symptoms of hay fever and have the advantage of causing less sedation than some of the older antihistamines. *Terfenadine* is now a Prescription Only Medicine (POM).

Astemizole has a long duration of action and requires only once-daily dosage, as do *cetirizine* and *loratadine*. Recommended doses should not be exceeded. For sale OTC, *astemizole, cetirizine* and *loratadine* can be recommended for children over 12 years of age. *Astemizole* has a long half-life and its full effects may take a day or longer to develop. This drug may be most effective when taken continously during the hay fever season.

While drowsiness is an extremely unlikely side-effect of any of the three drugs, patients might be well advised to try the treatment for a day before driving or operating machinery.

Cetirizine and *loratadine* may be recommended for other allergic disorders such as perennial rhinitis and urticaria, while currently *astemizole* is to be recommended for hay fever only.

Older antihistamines, such as *promethazine* and *diphenhydramine*, have a greater tendency to produce sedative effects. Indeed, both drugs are available in the UK in OTC products promoted for the management of temporary sleep disorders (see p. 269). The shorter half-life of *diphenhydramine* (5–8 hours compared to *promethazine*'s 8–12 hours) should mean less likelihood of a morning hangover/drowsiness effect.

Other older antihistamines are relatively less sedative, such as *chlorpheniramine* and *clemastine*. Patients may develop tolerance to their sedation effects. Anticholinergic activity is very much lower among the newer drugs compared to the older drugs.

Interactions

The potential sedative effects of older antihistamines are increased by alcohol, hypnotics, sedatives and anxiolytics. The alcohol content of some OTC medicines should be remembered.

The UK Committee on Safety of Medicines issued information on interactions between *terfenadine* and *astemizole* and other drugs in late 1992. Both drugs have the potential to induce ventricular arrhythmias. Concurrent administration with certain drugs predisposes to cardio-toxicity and *terfenadine* and *astemizole* should not be dispensed. The drugs involved are: *erythromycin, oral ketoconazole,* anti-arrhythmics, neuroleptics (e.g. *chlorpromazine*) tricyclic antidepressants (e.g. *amitriptyline*) and drugs which may cause electrolyte imbalance, such as diuretics. Patients should always be reminded not to exceed the recommended dose of these antihistamines. Terfenadine reverted to POM status in 1998 as a result of concerns about safety.

There have been isolated reports of an interaction between *phenytoin* and *chlorpheniramine*, in which the *phenytoin* levels were raised to toxic levels while the patients were taking *chlorpheniramine*. The mechanism is uncertain, but it has been suggested that antihistamines might inhibit liver metabolism of *phenytoin*. Antihistamines can antagonize the effects of *betahistine*.

Side effects

The major side effect of the older antihistamines is their potential to cause drowsiness. Their anticholinergic activity may result in a dry mouth, blurred vision, constipation and urinary retention. These effects will be increased if the patient is already taking another drug with anticholinergic effects (e.g. tricyclic antidepressants, neuroleptics).

At very high doses, antihistamines have central nervous system (CNS) excitatory rather than depressive effects. Such effects seem to be more likely to occur in children. At toxic levels, there have been reports of fits being induced. As a result, it has been suggested that antihistamines should be used with care in epileptic patients. However, this appears to be a largely theoretical risk.

Antihistamines are best avoided by patients with narrow- (closed-) angle glaucoma, since the anticholinergic effects produced can cause an increase in intra-ocular pressure. They should be used with caution in patients with liver disease or prostatic hypertrophy.

Interactions:
  alcohol
  hypnotics/anxiolytics
  sedatives (including barbiturates)
  phenytoin
  betahistine
  anticholinergics (tricyclics, *benzhexol*)
  erythromycin (interaction with *terfenadine* and *astemizole*)
  ketoconazole (interaction with *terfenadine* and *astemizole*)
  neuroleptics (e.g. *chlorpromazine*) (interaction with *terfenadine/
    astemizole*)
  tricyclic antidepressants
  anti-arrhythmics
  diuretics.
Side effects:
  drowsiness (driving, occupational hazard)
  constipation and anticholinergic effects.
Cautions:
  prostatic obstruction
  glaucoma.

Decongestants

Oral or topical decongestants may be used to reduce nasal congestion alone or in combination with an antihistamine. They can be useful in patients using a 'preventer' such as *cromoglycate, beclomethasone* or *flunisolide* where congestion can prevent the drug from reaching the nasal mucosa. Topical decongestants can cause rebound congestion, especially with prolonged use. They should not be used for more than a week. The decongestants are sympathomimetics such as *pseudoephedrine* and *phenylpropanolamine*. Their use, interactions and adverse effects are considered in the section on Colds and flu (see p. 17).

Eye drops containing an antihistamine and sympathomimetic combination are available and may be of value in troublesome eye symptoms, particularly when symptoms are intermittent. The sympathomimetic acts as a vasoconstrictor, reducing irritation and redness. Some patients find that the vasoconstrictor causes painful stinging when first applied. Eyedrops which contain a vasoconstrictor should not be used in patients who have glaucoma or who wear soft contact lenses.

Steroid nasal sprays

Beclomethasone nasal spray (aqueous pump rather than aerosol version) and *flunisolide* can be used for the treatment of seasonal allergic rhinitis.

A steroid nasal spray is the treatment of choice for moderate to severe nasal symptoms. The steroid acts to reduce inflammation which has occurred as a result of the allergen's action. Regular use is essential for full benefit to be obtained and treatment should be continued throughout the hay fever season. This needs to be explained carefully to the patient to ensure compliance. If symptoms of hay fever are already present, the patient needs to know that it is likely to take several days before the full treatment effect is reached.

Dryness and irritation of the nose and throat, and nosebleeds have occasionally been reported; otherwise side effects are rare. *Beclomethasone* or *flunisolide* nasal spray can be used in children over 12 years old and adults. They should not be recommended for pregnant women or for anyone with glaucoma.

Patients are sometimes alarmed by the term 'steroid', associating it with potent oral steroids and possible side effects. Therefore the pharmacist needs to take account of these concerns in explanations about the drug and how it works.

Sodium cromoglycate

This is available OTC as nasal drops or spray and as eye drops. An OTC nasal spray product containing *sodium cromoglycate* with a small amount of decongestant is available. The amount of decongestant is said to be too small to produce rebound congestion. *Cromoglycate* can be effective as a prophylactic if used correctly. It should be started at least a week before the hay fever season is likely to begin and then used continuously. There seem to be no significant side effects, although nasal irritation may occasionally occur.

Cromoglycate eye drops are effective for the treatment of eye symptoms which are not controlled by antihistamines. *Cromoglycate* should be used continously to obtain full benefit. The eye drops should be used four times a day. The eye drops contain the preservative *benzalkonium chloride* and should not be used by wearers of soft contact lenses.

Azelastine

This is available as a nasal spray and its active ingredient, the antihistamine *Azelastine*, has moved from POM to Pharmacy Medicine (P). The *British National Formulary* states it is 'Less effective than a *corticosteroid* nasal spray but probably more effective than *cromoglycate*', Its place in treatment is likely to be for mild and intermittent symptoms. The maximum treatment period is four weeks and it can be used in adults and children over 12 years of age. Advise the patient to keep the head upright during use to prevent the liquid trickling into the throat and causing an unpleasant taste.

Further advice

1 Car windows and air vents should be kept closed while driving. Otherwise a high pollen concentration inside the car can result.

2 Where house-dust mite is identified as a problem, regular cleaning of the house to maintain dust levels at a minimum can help. Special vacuum cleaners are now on sale which are claimed to be particularly effective.

Hay fever in practice

Case 1

A young man in his early twenties presents in late May. He asks what you can recommend for his runny nose, which he has had since the day before yesterday. On questioning, he tells you that his eyes have been itching a little and are slightly watery, that he has been sneezing and that his throat is dry. He has not had hay fever in the past. He will not be driving, but is a student at the local college and has exams coming up next week. He is not taking any medicines.

The pharmacist's view

This man is experiencing the classic symptoms of hay fever for the first time. The nasal symptoms are causing the most discomfort; he has rhinorrhoea rather than congestion so it would be reasonable to recommend an antihistamine, bearing in mind that he is sitting exams soon and so any preparation that might cause drowsiness is best avoided. His eyes are slightly irritated, but the symptoms are not very troublesome. You know that he is not taking any other medicines, so you could recommend *astemizole, loratadine* or *cetirizine*. If the symptoms are not better in a few days, he should see the doctor.

The doctor's view

Astemizole, loratadine or *cetirizine* would be a sensible first-line treatment. Even though they are generally non-sedating they can cause drowsiness in some patients. The student should be advised not to take his first dose just before the exam! If his symptoms do not settle, then referral is appropriate. He may benefit from *sodium cromoglycate* eye drops if his eye symptoms are not fully controlled by the antihistamine. It is often worthwhile trying an older antihistamine as an alternative because some people are unaffected by the sedative properties or become tolerant to them.

Case 2

A woman in her early thirties wants some advice. She tells you that she has hay fever and a blocked nose and is finding it difficult to breathe. You find out that she has had the symptoms for a few days; they have gradually got worse. She gets hay fever every summer and it is usually controlled by *chlorpheniramine* tablets, which she buys every year and which she is taking at the moment. As a child, she suffered quite badly from eczema and is still troubled by it occasionally. She tells you that she has been a little wheezy for the past day or so, but she does not have a cough, and has not coughed up any sputum. She is not taking any other medicines.

The pharmacist's view

This woman has a previous history of hay fever which has, until now, been dealt with adequately by *chlorpheniramine* tablets. Her symptoms have worsened over a period of a few days and she is now wheezing. It seems unlikely that she has a chest infection, which could have been a possible cause of the symptoms. She should be referred to the doctor at once since her symptoms suggest more serious implications such as asthma.

If the serious symptoms had not been present it would have been reasonable, because of the nasal symptoms and congestion, to suggest treatment with *beclomethasone* or *flunisolide* nasal spray, with an explanation that the full treatment effect would develop within 3–4 days.

The doctor's view

This woman should be referred to her doctor directly. She almost certainly has seasonal asthma. In addition to the hay fever treatment recommended by her phamacist it is likely that she would also benefit from a steroid inhaler such as *beclomethasone*. Depending on the severity of her symptoms she would probably be prescribed a β-agonist, such as a *salbutamol* inhaler, as well. This consultation is a complex one for a doctor to manage in the usual 10 minutes available in view of the time required for: information giving, explanation about the nature of the problem, the rationale for the treatments and the technique of using inhalers.

Respiratory symptoms for direct referral

Chest pain

Respiratory causes

A knife-like pain is characteristic of pleurisy. It is a localized pain which is aggravated by taking a breath or coughing. It is usually caused by a respiratory infection and may be associated with an underlying pneumonia.

Less commonly it may be caused by a pulmonary embolus (a blood clot which has lodged in a pulmonary artery after separating from a clot elsewhere in the circulation).

A similar pain to that experienced with pleurisy may arise from straining the muscles between the ribs following coughing. It may also occur with cracked or fractured ribs following injury or violent coughing. Another less common cause of pain is due to a pneumothorax where a small leak develops in the lung causing its collapse.

The upper front part of the chest may be very sore in the early stages of acute viral infections which cause inflammation of the trachea (tracheitis). Viral flu-like infections can be associated with non-specific muscular pain (myalgia).

Non-respiratory causes

Heartburn

This occurs when the acid contents of the stomach leak backwards into the oesophagus (gullet). The pain is described as a burning sensation which spreads upwards towards the throat. Occasionally it can be so severe as to mimic cardiac pain.

Cardiac pain

Cardiac pain typically presents as a tight, gripping, vice-like, dull pain which is felt centrally across the front of the chest. The pain may seem to move down one or both arms. Sometimes the pain spreads to the neck. When angina is present the pain is brought on by exercise and relieved by rest. When a coronary (coronary thrombosis, heart attack, myocardial infarction) occurs the pain is identical but more severe and prolonged. It may come on at rest.

Anxiety

This is a commonly seen cause of chest pain in general practice. The pain probably arises as a result of hyperventilation. Diagnosis can be difficult as the hyperventilation may not be obvious.

Shortness of breath

Shortness of breath may be a symptom of a cardiac or respiratory disorder. Differential diagnosis can be difficult. At one extreme the symptom can herald life-threatening problems and at the other a troublesome but non-serious disorder.

Respiratory causes

Asthma

Occasionally this may develop in later life, but it is most commonly seen in young children or young adults. The breathlessness is typically associated with a wheeze, although in mild cases the only symptom may be a recurrent nocturnal cough. Most asthmatics have normal breathing between attacks. The attacks are often precipitated by viral infections such as colds. Some are worsened in the hay fever season, others by animal fur or dust. The breathlessness is often worse at night.

Chronic bronchitis and emphysema

These disorders are usually caused by cigarette smoking and give rise to permanent breathlessness, especially on exertion, with a productive cough. The breathing worsens when an infective episode develops. At such times there is also an increase in coloured sputum production.

Cardiac causes

Heart failure

This may develop gradually or present acutely as an emergency (usually in the middle of the night). The former (congestive cardiac failure) may cause breathlessness on exertion. It is often associated with ankle swelling (oedema) and is most common in the elderly. The more sudden type is called acute left ventricular failure (LVF). The victim is woken by severe breathlessness and has to sit upright. There is often a cough present with clear frothy sputum.

Other causes

Hyperventilation syndrome

This occurs when the rate of breathing is too high for the bodily requirements. Paradoxically the subjective experience is that of breathlessness.
The sufferer complains of difficulty in taking in a deep breath. The
experience is frightening but harmless. It may be associated with other
symptoms such as tingling in the hands and feet, numbness around the
mouth, dizziness and various muscular aches. It may be caused by anxiety.

Wheezing

Wheezing sounds may be heard in the 'throat' region in upper respiratory
infections and are of little consequence. They are to be differentiated
from wheezing emanating from the lungs. In these latter situations there
is usually some difficulty in breathing.

Wheezy bronchitis

Wheezing occurs in infants with wheezy bronchitis. It is caused by a
viral infection and is completely different from chronic bronchitis seen
in adults. The infection is self-limiting but requires accurate diagnosis.
Children who have a history of recurrent wheezy bronchitis are more
likely to develop asthma.

Asthma

Wheezing is a common feature of asthma, and accompanies the shortness
of breath. However, in very mild asthma it is not obvious and may
present with just a cough. At the other extreme an asthma attack can
be so severe that so little air moves in and out of the lungs that there is
no audible wheeze.

Cardiac

Wheezing may be a symptom associated with the shortness of breath in
heart failure.

Sputum

Sputum may be described as thick or thin and clear or coloured. It is a
substance coughed up from the lungs and is not to be confused with
saliva or nasal secretions.

Bronchitis

Clear thick sputum may be coughed up in chronic bronchitis or by regular cigarette smokers. It has a mucoid nature and may be described as white, grey or clear with black particles. Chronic bronchitics are prone to recurrent infective exacerbations during which sputum production increases and turns yellow or green.

Pneumonia
Coloured mucoid sputum may be present in other lung infections such as pneumonia. Rusty-coloured sputum is characteristic of pneumococcal (lobar) pneumonia.

Cardiac
Clear thin (serous) sputum may be a feature of heart failure (LVF). The sputum forms as a result of pulmonary oedema which characteristically awakens the patient in the night with shortness of breath.

Haemoptysis
The presence of blood in sputum is always alarming. It often results from a broken capillary caused by coughing and is harmless. However, it can be a symptom of serious disease such as lung cancer or pulmonary tuberculosis (TB) and should always be referred for further investigation. Occasionally blood is coughed up after a nose bleed and is of no consequence.

Gastrointestinal Tract Problems

Mouth ulcers

Mouth ulcers are extremely common, affecting as many as one in two of the population and they are a recurrent problem in some people. They are classified as aphthous (minor or major) or herpetiform ulcers. Most cases (more than three-quarters) are minor aphthous ulcers, which are self-limiting. Ulcers may be due to a variety of causes including infection, trauma and drug allergy. However, occasionally mouth ulcers appear as a symptom of serious disease such as carcinoma. The pharmacist should be aware of the signs and characteristics which indicates more serious conditions.

> **What you need to know**
>
> Age
>   Child, adult
> Nature of the ulcers
>   Size, appearance, location, number
> Duration
> Previous history
> Other symptoms
> Medication

Significance of questions and answers

Age
Patients may describe a history of recurrent ulceration which began in childhood and has continued ever since. Minor aphthous ulcers are more common in women and occur most often between the ages of 10 and 40.

Nature of the ulcers
Minor aphthous ulcers usually occur in crops of one to five. The lesions may be up to 5 mm in diameter and appear as a white or yellowish centre with an inflamed red outer edge. Common sites are the tongue margin and inside the lips and cheeks.

Other types of recurrent mouth ulcer include major aphthous and herpetiform. Major aphthous ulcers are uncommon severe variants of the minor ones. The ulcers, which may be as large as 30 mm in diameter, can occur in crops of up to 10. Sites involved are the lips, cheeks, tongue, pharynx and palate. They are more common in sufferers of ulcerative colitis.

Herpetiform ulcers are more numerous, smaller and in addition to the sites involved with aphthous ulcers, may affect the floor of the mouth and the gums.

Systemic conditions such as Behçet's syndrome and erythema multi-forme may produce mouth ulcers, but other symptoms would generally be present (see below).

Duration

Minor aphthous ulcers usually heal in less than a week; major aphthous ulcers take longer (10–30 days). Where herpetiform ulcers occur, fresh crops of ulcers tend to appear before the original crop has healed, which may lead patients to think that the ulceration is continuous.

Oral cancer

Any mouth ulcer which has persisted for longer than 3 weeks requires immediate referral to the dentist or doctor because an ulcer of such long duration may indicate serious pathology such as carcinoma. Most oral cancers are squamous cell carcinomas, of which one in three affects the lip and one in four affects the tongue. The development of a cancer may be preceded by a premalignant lesion, including erythroplasia (red) and leucoplakia (white), or a speckled leucoplakia. The key point to raise suspicion would be a lesion which had lasted for several weeks or longer. Oral cancer is more common in smokers than non-smokers.

Previous history

There is often a family history of mouth ulcers (estimated to be present in one in three cases). Minor aphthous ulcers often recur, with the same characteristic features of size, numbers, appearance and duration before healing. The appearance of these ulcers may follow trauma to the inside of the mouth or tongue, such as biting the inside of the cheek while chewing food.

Ill-fitting dentures may produce ulceration and, if this is suspected as a cause, the patient should be referred back to the dentist so that the dentures can be re-fitted. However, trauma is not always a feature of the history and the cause of minor aphthous ulcers remains unclear despite extensive investigation.

In women, minor aphthous ulcers often precede the start of the menstrual period. The occurrence of ulcers may cease after pregnancy, suggesting hormonal involvement. Stress and emotional factors at work or home may precipitate a recurrence or a delay in healing but do not seem to be causative.

Deficiency of iron, folate or vitamin B_{12} may be a contributory factor in aphthous ulcers and may also lead to glossitis (a condition where the tongue becomes sore, red and smooth) and angular stomatitis (where the corners of the mouth become sore, cracked and red).

Food allergy is occasionally the causative factor and it is worth enquiring whether the appearance of ulcers is associated with particular foods.

Other symptoms

The severe pain associated with major aphthous or herpetiform ulcers may mean that the patient finds it difficult to eat and, as a consequence, weight loss may occur. Weight loss would therefore be an indication for referral.

In most cases of recurrent mouth ulcers the disease eventually burns itself out over a period of several years. Occasionally, as in Behcet's syndrome, there is progression with involvement of sites other than the mouth. Most commonly the vulva, vagina and the eyes are affected, with genital ulceration and iritis (see p. 230).

Behçet's syndrome can be confused with erythema multiforme although in the latter there is usually a distinctive rash present on the skin. Erythema multiforme is sometimes precipitated by an infection or drugs (e.g. sulphonamides or barbiturates).

Mouth ulcers may be associated with inflammatory bowel disorders or with coeliac disease. Therefore, if persistent or recurrent diarrhoea is present then referral is essential.

Patients reporting any of these symptoms should be referred to their doctor.

Rarely, ulcers may be associated with disorders of the blood including anaemia, abnormally low white cell count or leukaemia. It would be expected that in these situations there would be other signs of illness present and the sufferer would present directly to the doctor.

Medication

The pharmacist should establish the identity of any current medication, since mouth ulcers may be produced as a side effect of drug therapy. Drugs which have been reported to cause the problem include *aspirin* and other non-steroidal anti-inflammatory agents, cytotoxic drugs and *sulphasalazine*. Radiotherapy may also induce mouth ulcers. It is worth asking about herbal medicines because *feverfew* (used for migraine) can cause mouth ulcers.

It would also be useful to ask the patient about any treatments tried either previously or on this occasion and the degree or relief obtained. The pharmacist can then recommend an alternative product where appropriate.

Treatment timescale

If there is no improvement after a week, the patient should see the doctor.

Management

Symptomatic treatment of minor aphthous ulcers can be recommended by the pharmacist, and can help to relieve discomfort and pain. Active ingredients include antiseptics, local anaesthetics and anti-inflammatory agents. Commonly used preparations include gels, liquids, mouthwashes, pastilles and tablets. Gels and liquids may be more accurately applied using a cotton bud or cotton wool, providing the ulcer is readily accessible. Mouthwashes can be useful where ulcers are difficult to reach.

Local anaesthetics (e.g. *lignocaine, benzocaine*)

Local anaesthetic gels form one of the most popular treatments for mouth ulcers. Although they are effective in producing pain relief, maintenance of gels and liquids in contact with the ulcer surface is difficult. Reapplication of the preparation may be made when necessary. Tablets and pastilles can be kept in contact with the ulcer by the tongue and can be very useful when just one or two ulcers are present. Any preparation containing a local anaesthetic becomes difficult to use when the lesions are located in inaccessible parts of the mouth.

Both *lignocaine* and *benzocaine* have been reported to produce sensitization, but cross-sensitivity seems to be rare, probably because the two agents are from different chemical groupings. Thus, if a patient has experienced a reaction to one agent in the past, the alternative could be tried.

Topical analgesic (*choline salicylate*)

Choline salicylate dental gel is frequently recommended for the symptomatic treatment of mouth ulcers. Again, while it is effective in relieving pain, retention of the gel in contact with the ulcer is difficult and reapplication will be necessary.

Although aspirin is no longer recommended for children under 12 years old because of possible links with Reye's syndrome, *choline salicylate* dental gel produces low levels of *salicylate* and can, therefore, be recommended for children.

Antibacterials (e.g. *chlorhexidine gluconate, cetylpyridinium chloride, povidone-iodine*)

The rationale for the use of antibacterial agents in the treatment of mouth ulcers is that secondary bacterial infection frequently occurs. Such infection can increase discomfort and delay healing. Preparations available include mouthwashes, pastilles and pellets. Mouthwashes are especially useful where there are several lesions, or where ulcers are located in parts of the mouth which are difficult to reach. Products containing *chlorhexidine* may discolour the tongue and teeth.

Anti-inflammatory agents (e.g. *hydrocortisone, triamcinolone, benzydamine, carbenoxolone*)

Hydrocortisone and *triamcinolone* act locally on the ulcer to reduce inflammation and pain. The former is available as pellets, the latter in a protective paste (see below). To exert its effect, a pellet must be held in close proximity to the ulcer until dissolved. This can be difficult when the ulcer is in an inaccessible spot. One pellet is used four times a day. The pharmacist should explain to the patient that the pellets should not be sucked, but dissolved in contact with the ulcer. When the deregulation of *hydrocortisone* oral pellets from prescription only status was agreed in 1994, the importance of limiting the treatment period was highlighted to ensure early referral where an ulcer does not heal and treatment is restricted to 5 days.

Benzydamine is available as a mouthwash and can be useful when ulcers are located in inaccessible areas, or where there are several lesions. *Benzydamine* has been reported to cause numbness and tingling of the mouth as adverse effects in a small number of users. *Benzydamine* mouthwash is not recommended for children under 12 years of age.

Carbenoxolone is available as an oral gel, which is applied in a thick layer to the ulcers after meals and before going to bed.

Protective agents

Carmellose dental paste forms a protective mechanical barrier when applied to ulcers, and can be reapplied as needed. The preparation is even more effective when the corticosteroid *triamcinolone* is added, particularly when used during the prodromal phase. (Before the ulcer appears the affected area feels sensitive and tingling and this is termed the prodromal phase.) *Carmellose dental paste* with the steroid *triamcinolone* is a 'pharmacy only' medicine with a restricted treatment period of up to 5 days. The preparation is considered by some experts to be the most effective available for the treatment of mouth ulcers.

Other substances

Alum was a traditional remedy for mouth ulcers because of its astringent action. However, far from aiding healing, it is now known to have the potential to actually damage tissues, thus delaying healing.

Tincture of myrrh has been used in the past as an ingredient of mouth-washes in the treatment of mouth ulcers. As more effective treatments are now available, its use has been largely superseded.

Mouth ulcers in practice

Case 1

Anthony Jarvis, a man aged in his early fifities, asks you to recommend something for painful mouth ulcers. On questioning, he tells you that he has two ulcers at the moment and has occasionally suffered from the problem over many years. Usually he gets one or two ulcers inside the cheek or lips and they last for about a week. Mr Jarvis is not taking any medicines and has no other symptoms. You ask to see the lesions and note that there are two small white patches, each with an angry-looking red border. One ulcer is located on the edge of the tongue, the other inside the cheek. Mr Jarvis cannot remember any trauma or injury to the mouth and has had the ulcers for a couple of days. He tells you that he has used pain-killing gels in the past and they provided some relief.

The pharmacist's view

From what he has told you, it would be reasonable to assume that Mr Jarvis suffers from recurrent minor aphthous ulcers. Treatment with *hydrocortisone* pellets (one pellet dissolved in contact with the ulcers four times a day), with *triamcinolone* in *carmellose dental paste*, or with a local anaesthetic or analgesic gel applied when needed, would help relieve discomfort until the ulcers healed. Mr Jarvis should see his doctor if the ulcers have not healed within 3 weeks.

The doctor's view

Mr Jarvis is most likely suffering from recurrent aphthous ulceration. As always, it is worthwhile enquiring about his general health, checking in particular that he does not have a recurrent bowel upset or weight loss. These ulcers can be helped by a topical steroid preparation.

Case 2

One of your counter assistants asks you to recommend a strong treatment for mouth ulcers for a woman who has already tried several treatments. The woman tells you that she has a troublesome ulcer which has persisted for a few weeks. She has used some pastilles containing a local anaesthetic and an antiseptic mouthwash but with no improvement.

The pharmacist's view

This woman should be advised to see her doctor for further investigation. The ulcer has been present for several weeks, with no sign of improvement, suggesting the possibility of a serious cause.

The doctor's view

Referral is correct. It is likely that the doctor will refer her to an oral surgeon for further assessment and probable biopsy as the ulcer could be malignant. Cancer of the mouth accounts for approximately 2% of all cancers of the body in Britain. It is most common after the sixth decade and is more common in men, especially pipe or cigar smokers. Cancer of the mouth is most often found on the tongue or lower lip. It may be painless initially.

Heartburn

Symptoms of heartburn are caused when there is reflux of gastric contents, particularly acid, into the oesophagus, which irritate the sensitive mucosal surface (oesophagitis). Patients will often describe the symptoms of heartburn; typically a burning discomfort/pain felt in the stomach passing upwards behind the breastbone (retrosternally). By careful questioning, the pharmacist can distinguish conditions which are potentially more serious.

What you need to know

Age
   Adult, child
Symptoms
   Heartburn
   Difficulty in swallowing
   Flatulence
Associated factors
   Pregnancy
   Precipitating factors
   Relieving factors
   Weight
   Smoking habit
   Eating
Medication
   Medicines tried already
   Other medicines being taken

Significance of questions and answers

Age

The symptoms of reflux and oesophagitis occur more commonly in patients aged over 55. Heartburn is not a condition normally experienced in childhood, although symptoms can occur in young adults and particularly in pregnant women. Children with symptoms of heartburn should therefore be referred to their doctor.

Symptoms/associated factors

A burning discomfort is experienced in the upper part of the stomach in the midline (epigastrium) and the burning feeling tends to move upwards behind the breastbone (retrosternally). The pain may be felt only in the lower retrosternal area or on occasion be felt right up to the throat, causing an acid taste in the mouth.

Deciding whether or not someone is suffering from heartburn can be greatly helped by enquiring about precipitating or aggravating factors. Heartburn is often brought on by bending or lying down. It is more likely to occur in the overweight and can be aggravated by a recent increase in weight. It is also more likely to occur after a large meal. It can be aggravated and even caused by belching. Many people develop a nervous habit of swallowing to clear the throat. Each time this occurs, air is taken down into the stomach, which becomes distended. This causes discomfort which is relieved by belching but which in turn can be associated with acid reflux.

Severe pain

Sometimes the pain can come on suddenly and severely and even radiate to the back and arms. In this situation differentiation of symptoms is difficult as the pain can mimic a heart attack and urgent medical referral is essential. Sometimes patients who have been admitted to hospital apparently suffering a heart attack are found to have oesophagitis instead.

For further discussion about causes of chest pain, see p. 52.

Difficulty in swallowing (dysphagia)

This must always be regarded as a serious symptom. The difficulty may either be discomfort as food or drink is swallowed or a sensation of food or liquids sticking in the gullet. Both require referral (see *When to refer* section). It is possible that discomfort may be secondary to oesophagitis from acid reflux (gastro-oesophageal reflux disease, GORD), especially when it occurs whilst swallowing hot drinks or irritant fluids (e.g. alcohol or fruit juice). A history of a sensation that food sticks as it is swallowed or that it does not seem to pass directly into the stomach (dysphagia) is an indication for immediate referral. It may be due to obstruction of the oesophagus, for example by a tumour.

Regurgitation

Regurgitation can be associated with difficulty in swallowing. It occurs when recently eaten food sticks in the oesophagus and is regurgitated without passing into the stomach. This is due to a mechanical blockage in the oesophagus. This can be caused by a cancer or, more fortunately, by less serious conditions such as a peptic stricture. A peptic stricture is caused by long-standing acid reflux with oesophagitis. The continual inflammation of the oesophagus causes scarring. Scars contract and can therefore cause narrowing of the oesophagus. This can be treated by dilatation using a fibre optic endoscope. However, medical examination and further investigations are necessary to determine the cause of regurgitation.

Pregnancy

It has been estimated that as many as half of all pregnant women suffer from heartburn. Pregnant women aged over 30 are more likely to suffer from the problem. The symptoms are caused by an increase in intra-abdominal pressure and incompetence of the lower oesophageal sphincter. It is thought that hormonal influences, particularly progesterone, are important in the lowering of sphincter pressure. Heartburn often begins in mid- to late pregnancy, but may happen at any stage. The problem may sometimes be associated with stress.

Medication

The pharmacist should establish the identity of any medication which has been tried to treat the symptoms. Any other medication being taken by the patient should also be identified; some drugs can cause the symptoms of heartburn, for example, anticholinergic agents such as *hyoscine* and drugs with anticholinergic actions such as tricyclic antidepressants and phenothiazines. Calcium channel blockers, nitrates, *theophylline* and *aminophylline* can also aggravate heartburn, as can caffeine.

Failure to respond to antacids and pain radiating to the arms could mean that the pain is not caused by acid reflux. Acid reflux is still a possibility but other causes such as ischaemic heart disease and gall bladder disease have to be considered.

When to refer

Failure to respond to antacids
Pain radiating to arms
Difficulty in swallowing
Regurgitation
Long duration
Increasing severity
Children

Treatment timescale

If symptoms have not responded to treatment after 1 week the patient should see the doctor.

Management

The symptoms of heartburn respond well to treatments which are available over the counter (OTC) and there is also a role for the pharmacist to offer practical advice about measures to prevent recurrence of the problem.

Antacids

These can be effective in controlling the symptoms of heartburn and reflux, more so in combination with an alginate. Choice of antacid can be made by the pharmacist using the same guidelines as in the section on indigestion (see p. 79). Preparations which are high in sodium should be avoided by anyone on a sodium-restricted diet (e.g. those with congestive heart failure or kidney or liver problems).

Alginates

Alginates form a raft which sits on the surface of the stomach contents and prevents reflux. Some alginate-based products are high in sodium because their formulation includes *sodium bicarbonate*. The function of the *sodium bicarbonate*, in addition to its antacid action, is to cause the release of carbon dioxide gas in the stomach, enabling the 'raft' to float on top of the stomach contents. If a preparation low in sodium is required, the pharmacist can recommend one containing *potassium bicarbonate* instead. Alginate products with a low sodium content are useful for the treatment of heartburn in patients on a restricted sodium diet (see above).

H₂ antagonists (*cimetidine, famotidine, ranitidine*)

These H$_2$ antagonists have been deregulated from prescription only control for the short-term treatment (up to 2 weeks) of dyspepsia, hyperacidity and heartburn (see also p. 82). The 2-week treatment limit is intended to ensure that patients do not continuously self-medicate for long periods. Pharmacists and their staff can ask whether use has been continuous or intermittent when a repeat purchase request is made. The H$_2$ antagonists have both a longer duration of action (up to 8–9 hours) and a longer onset of action than antacids.

Where food is known to precipitate symptoms, the H$_2$ antagonist should be taken an hour before food. H$_2$ antagonists are also effective for prophylaxis of nocturnal heartburn. Headache, dizziness, diarrhoea and skin rashes have been reported as adverse effects but they are not common.

Preparations containing *cimetidine, famotidine* and *ranitidine* have been widely advertised to the public. Such advertising is bound to result in many requests to purchase a named product and pharmacists and their staff rightly feel it is their responsibility to ensure that the product is appropriate. Carefully phrased questions are required, perhaps with an explanation of why the information is needed. Manufacturers state that patients should not take OTC *cimetidine*, *famotidine* or *ranitidine* without checking with their doctor if they are taking other prescribed medicines.

Cimetidine

Cimetidine can be sold OTC at a maximum dose of 200 mg and maximum daily dose of 800 mg. The drug binds to microsomal cytochrome P450 in the liver and inhibits the normal operation of the enzyme system, increasing the levels of some drugs. As a result *cimetidine* has a number of significant interactions with other drugs, including *theophylline*, resulting in toxic levels of *theophylline*. Other important concurrent drugs to avoid are *warfarin* and *phenytoin*. The *British National Formulary* appendix on drug interactions gives further information.

Famotidine

Famotidine does not affect the cytochrome P450 system and therefore does not cause the same range of interactions as *cimetidine*. The drug is licensed for OTC use at a maximum dose of 10 mg and maximum daily dose of 20 mg.

Ranitidine

Ranitidine is licensed for OTC use in a dose of 75 mg with a maximum of 300 mg in 24 hours. *Ranitidine* does not affect the cytochrome P450 system.

Practical points

Obesity

If the patient is overweight, weight reduction should be advised. Most patients will find that their symptoms will cease when they attain their ideal weight.

Food

Small meals, eaten frequently, are better than large meals as reducing the amount of food in the stomach reduces gastric distension which helps to prevent reflux. Gastric emptying is slowed when there is a large volume of food in the stomach; this can also aggravate symptoms. Evening meal is best taken several hours before going to bed.

Posture

Bending, stooping and even slumping in an armchair can provoke symptoms and should be avoided where possible. It is better to squat rather than bend down. Since the symptoms are often worse when the patient lies down, raising the head of the bed may help. Using extra pillows is often recommended but this is not as effective as raising the head of the bed. The reason for this is that using extra pillows raises only the upper part of the body, with bending at the waist, which can result in increased pressure on the stomach contents.

Clothing

Tight, constricting clothing, especially waistbands and belts, can be an aggravating factor and should be avoided.

Other aggravating factors

Smoking, alcohol, caffeine, chocolate and fatty foods can all make the oesophageal sphincter less competent by reducing its pressure and therefore contribute to symptoms. The pharmacist is in a good position to offer advice about how to stop smoking, offering a smoking cessation product where appropriate. The knowledge that the discomfort of heartburn will be reduced can be a motivating factor in giving up cigarettes.

Heartburn in practice

Case 1

Mrs Amy Beston is a woman aged about 50 who wants some advice about a stomach problem. On questioning, you find out that sometimes she gets a burning sensation just above the breastbone and that she feels the burning in her throat, sometimes with a bitter taste as if some food has been brought back up. She has been having the problem for a week or two and has not yet tried to treat it. Mrs Beston is not taking any medicines from the doctor. To your experienced eye this lady is at least a stone overweight. You ask Mrs Beston if the symptoms are worse at any particular time and she says they are worst shortly after going to bed at night.

The pharmacist's view

This woman has many of the classic symptoms of heartburn; pain in the restrosternal region and reflux. The problem is worse at night after going to bed, as is common in heartburn. Mrs Beston has been experiencing the symptoms for about 2 weeks and is not taking any medicines from the doctor.

It would be reasonable to advise the use of an alginate antacid product about an hour after meals and before going to bed, or an H_2 antagonist. Practical advice could include the tactful suggestion that Mrs Beston's symptoms would be improved if she lost weight. Advice on healthy eating and contact with a local Weight Watchers group could be given. Mrs Beston could also try raising the head of the bed or using extra pillows at bedtime, wearing loose-fitting clothes, cutting down on tea, coffee and, if she smokes, on smoking. This is a long list of potential lifestyle changes. It might be a good idea to explain the contributory factors to Mrs Beston and negotiate with her as to which one she will begin with. Success is more likely to be achieved and sustained if changes are introduced one at a time.

Menopausal women are more prone to heartburn and weight gain at the time of the menopause will exacerbate the problem.

The doctor's view

The advice given by the pharmacist is sensible. Acid reflux is the most likely explanation for her symptoms. It is not clear from the presentation whether she was seeking medication or simply asking for an opinion about the cause of her symptoms, or both. It is always helpful to explore a patient's expectations in order to produce an effective outcome to a consultation. In this instance the interchange between the pharmacist and Mrs Beston is complex as a large amount of information needs to be given, both explaining the cause of the symptoms (providing an understandable description of oesphagus, stomach, acid reflux and oesophagitis) and advising about treatment and lifestyle. It is often sensible to offer a follow-up discussion to check on progress and reinforce advice. If her heartburn was not improving it would provide an opportunity to recommend referral to her doctor.

The doctor's next step would be very much dependent on this information. If a clear story of heartburn caused by acid reflux was obtained, then reinforcement of the pharmacist's advice concerning posture, weight, diet, smoking and alcohol would be appropriate. If medication was requested, antacids or alginates could be tried. If the symptoms were severe, an H_2 antagonist or *omeprazole* would be treatment options. An alternative would be *cisapride*, which affects the motility of the stomach and intestines. *Cisapride* causes increased oesophageal sphincter pressure, increased gastric emptying, reduced gastric acidity and is about as effective as *ranitidine* or *cimetidine* in mild to moderate reflux.

Case 2

You have been asked to recommend a 'strong' mixture for heartburn for Harry Groves, a local man in his late fifties who works in a nearby warehouse. Mr Groves tell you that he has been getting terrible heartburn for which his doctor prescribed some mixture about a week ago. You remember dispensing a prescription for a liquid alginate preparation. The bottle is now empty and the problem is no better. When asked if he can point to where the pain is, Mr Groves gestures across his chest and clenches his fist when describing the pain, which he says feels 'heavy'. You ask whether the pain ever moves and Mr Groves tells you that sometimes it goes to his neck and jaw. Mr Groves is a smoker and is not taking any other medicines. When asked if the pain worsens when bending or lying down, Mr Groves says it does not, but he tells you he usually gets the pain when he is at work, especially on busy days.

The pharmacist's view

This man should see his doctor immediately. The symptoms he has described are not those which would be typical of heartburn. In addition, he has been taking an alginate preparation which has been ineffective. Mr Groves' symptoms give cause for concern; the 'heartburn' is associated with effort at work and its location and radiation suggest a more serious cause.

The doctor's view

Mr Groves' story is suggestive of angina. He should be advised to contact his doctor immediately. The doctor would require more details about the pain, such as duration and whether or not the pain can come on without any exertion. If the periods of pain were frequent, prolonged and unrelieved by rest it would be usual to arrange immediate hospital admission as the picture sounds like unstable or crescendo angina.

If an urgent inpatient referral is not required, the doctor would carry out a fuller assessment which would usually include an examination, ECG (electrocardiogram), urine analysis and blood test. This in turn could lead to medication, for example *aspirin* or GTN (glyceryl trinitrate), possibly a long-acting nitrate (*isosorbide dinitrate*), perhaps a beta-blocker and/or calcium channel blocker being prescribed and an urgent outpatient referral to a cardiologist. Mr Groves would be strongly advised to stop smoking.

More detailed tests are likely to be arranged in hospital. These would probably include an exercise cardiogram and an angiogram. This latter test allows visualization of the blood vessels supplying the heart muscle and assessment of whether surgery would be advisable.

Indigestion

Indigestion (dyspepsia) is commonly presented in community pharmacies and is often self-diagnosed by patients, who use the term to include anything from pain in the chest and upper abdomen to lower abdominal symptoms. Many patients use the terms indigestion and heartburn interchangeably. The pharmacist must establish whether such a self-diagnosis is correct and exclude the possibility of serious disease.

What you need to know

Symptoms
Age
  Adult, child
Duration of symptoms
Previous history
Details of pain
  Where is the pain?
  What is its nature?
  Is it associated with food?
  Is the pain constant or colicky?
  Are there any aggravating or relieving factors?
  Does the pain move to anywhere else?
Associated symptoms
  Loss of appetite
  Weight loss
  Nausea/vomiting
  Alteration in bowel habit
Diet
  Any recent change of diet?
  Alcohol consumption
Smoking habit
Medication
  Medicines already tried
  Other medicines being taken

Significance of questions and answers

Symptoms

The symptoms of typical indigestion include poorly localized upper abdominal (the area between the belly button and the breastbone) discomfort which may be brought on by particular foods, excess food, alcohol or medication (e.g. *aspirin*).

Age

Indigestion is rare in children, who should be referred to the doctor. Abdominal pain, however, is a common symptom in children and is often associated with an infection. Over-the-counter (OTC) treatment is not appropriate for abdominal pain of unknown cause and referral to the doctor would be advisable.

Be cautious when dealing with first-time indigestion in older patients (aged 50 or over). Gastric cancer, while rare in young patients, is more likely to occur in those aged 50 and over. Careful history-taking is therefore of paramount importance here.

Duration/previous history

Indigestion which is persistent or recurrent should be referred to the doctor, after considering the information gained from questioning. Any patient with a previous history of the symptom which has not responded to treatment, or which has worsened, should be referred.

Details of pain/associated symptoms

If the pharmacist can obtain a good description of the pain then the decision whether to advise treatment or referral is much easier. A few medical conditions which may present as 'indigestion' but which require referral are described below.

Ulcer

Ulcers may occur in the stomach (gastric ulcer) or in the first part of the small intestine leading from the stomach (duodenal ulcer). Duodenal ulcers are more common and have different symptoms from gastric ulcers. Typically the pain of a duodenal ulcer is localized to the upper abdomen, slightly to the right of the midline. It is often possible to point to the site of pain with a single finger. The pain is dull and is most likely to occur when the stomach is empty, especially at night. It is relieved by food (although it may be aggravated by fatty foods) and antacids.

The pain of a gastric ulcer is in the same area but less well localized. It is often aggravated by food and may be associated with nausea and vomiting. Appetite is usually reduced and the symptoms are persistent and severe. Both types of ulcer may be exacerbated or precipitated by smoking and non-steroidal anti-inflammatory drugs (NSAIDs).

Gallstones

Single or multiple stones can form in the gall bladder, which is situated beneath the liver. The gall bladder stores bile. It periodically contracts to squirt bile through a narrow tube (bile duct) into the duodenum to aid digestion of food, especially fat. Stones can become temporarily stuck in the opening to the bile duct as the gall bladder contracts. This causes severe pain (biliary colic) in the upper abdomen below the right rib margin. Sometimes this pain can be confused with that of a duodenal ulcer. Biliary colic may be precipitated by a fatty meal.

Gastro-oesophageal reflux

When a person eats, food passes down the gullet (oesophagus) and into the stomach. Acid is produced by the stomach to aid digestion. The lining of the stomach is resistant to the irritant effects of acid, whereas the lining of the oesophagus is readily irritated by acid. A sphincter (valve) system operates between the stomach and the oesophagus preventing reflux of stomach contents.

When this 'valve system' is weak, for example in the presence of a hiatus hernia, or where sphincter muscle tone is reduced by drugs such as anticholinergics, *theophylline* and calcium channel blockers, the acid contents of the stomach can leak 'backwards' into the oesophagus. The symptoms arising are typically described as heartburn but many patients use the terms heartburn and indigestion interchangeably. Heartburn is a pain arising in the upper abdomen passing upwards behind the breastbone. It is often precipitated by a large meal, or by bending and lying down. Heartburn can be treated by the pharmacist but sometimes requires referral (see p. 68).

Irritable bowel syndrome

This is a common, non-serious but troublesome condition in which symptoms are caused by colon spasm (also see p. 112). There is usually an alteration in bowel habit, often with alternating constipation and diarrhoea. The diarrhoea is typically worse first thing in the morning. Pain is usually present. It is often lower abdominal (below and to the right or left of the belly button) but it may be upper and therefore confused with indigestion. Any persistent alteration in normal bowel habit is an indication for referral.

Atypical angina

Angina is usually experienced as a tight painful constricting band across the middle of the chest. Atypical angina pain may be felt in the lower chest or upper abdomen. It is likely to be precipitated by exercise or exertion. If this occurs then referral is necessary.

More serious disorders

Persisting upper abdominal pain, especially when associated with anorexia and unexplained weight loss, may herald an underlying cancer of the stomach or pancreas. Ulcers sometimes start bleeding which may present with blood in the vomit (haematemesis) or in the stool (melaena). In the latter the stool becomes tarry and black. Urgent referral is necessary.

Diet

Fatty foods and alcohol can cause indigestion, aggravate ulcers and precipitate biliary colic.

Smoking habit

Smoking predisposes to, and may cause, indigestion and ulcers. Ulcers heal more slowly and relapse more often during treatment in smokers. The pharmacist is in a good position to offer advice on smoking cessation, perhaps with a recommendation to use nicotine replacement therapy in the form of patches or gum.

Medication

Medicines already tried

Anyone who has tried one or more antacids without improvement or whose initial improvement in symptoms is not maintained should see the doctor.

Other medicines being taken

Gastrointestinal (GI) side effects can be caused by many drugs, so it is important for the pharmacist to ascertain any medication which the patient is taking.

Non-steroidal anti-inflammatory agents (NSAIDs) such as *ibuprofen, indomethacin* and *piroxicam* have been implicated in the causation of ulcers and bleeding ulcers. Sometimes these drugs cause indigestion. Elderly patients are particularly prone to such problems and pharmacists should bear this in mind. Severe or prolonged indigestion in any patient taking a NSAID is an indication for referral. Particular care is needed in elderly patients, when referral is always advisable.

Over-the-counter medicines also require consideration; *aspirin, ibuprofen* and *iron* are among those which may produce symptoms of indigestion. Some drugs may interact with antacids; these include antibiotics (the absorption of tetracyclines, *pivampcillin* and *ketoconazole* my be reduced if taken at the same time as antacids) and iron preparations. Absorption of *cimetidine*, *chlorpromazine* and *diflunisal* may also be reduced. Taking the doses of antacids and other drugs at least 1 hour apart should minimize the interaction.

Treatment timescale

If symptoms have not improved within 5 days the patient should see the doctor.

Management

Once the pharmacist has excluded serious disease, treatment of dyspepsia with antacids or an H_2 antagonist may be recommended and is likely to be effective. The preparation chosen should be selected on the basis of the individual patient's symptoms. Smoking, alcohol and fatty meals can all aggravate symptoms, so the pharmacist can advise appropriately.

Antacids

In general, liquids are more effective antacids than are solids; they are easier to take, work more quickly and have a greater neutralizing capacity. Their small particle size allows a large surfce area to be in contact with the gastric contents. Some patients find tablets more convenient and these should be well chewed before swallowing for the best effect. It might be appropriate for the patient to have both; the liquid could be taken before and after working hours while the tablets could be taken during the day for convenience. Antacids are best taken about an hour after a meal because the rate of gastric emptying has then slowed and the antacid will therefore remain in the stomach for longer. Taken at this time, antacids may act for up to 3 hours compared to only half an hour to an hour if taken before meals.

Sodium bicarbonate

This is the only absorbable antacid that is useful in practice. It is water soluble, acts quickly, is an effective neutralizer of acid and has a short duration of action. It is often included in OTC formulations in order to give a fast-acting effect, in combination with longer-acting agents. However, antacids containing *sodium bicarbonate* should be avoided in patients if sodium intake should be restricted (e.g. in patients with congestive heart failure). The contents of OTC products should therefore be carefully scrutinized and pharmacists should be aware of the constituents of some of the traditional formulary preparations. For example, *magnesium trisilicate mixture* contains *sodium bicarbonate* and is therefore relatively high in sodium. The relative sodium contents of different antacids can be found in the *British National Formulary*. In addition, long-term use of *sodium bicarbonate* may lead to systemic alkalosis and renal damage. In short-term use, however, it can be a valuable and effective antacid. Its use is more appropriate in acute rather than chronic dyspepsia.

Aluminium and magnesium salts (e.g. *aluminium hydroxide, magnesium trisilicate*)

Aluminium-based antacids are effective; they tend to be constipating and this can be a useful effect in patients if there is slight diarrhoea. Conversely, the use of aluminium antacids is best avoided in anyone who is constipated and in elderly patients, who have a tendency to be so. Magnesium salts are more potent acid neutralizers than aluminium. They tend to cause osmotic diarrhoea as a result of the formation of insoluble magnesium salts and are therefore useful in patients who are slightly constipated. Combination products containing aluminium and magnesium salts cause minimum bowel disturbance and are therefore valuable preparations for recommendation by the pharmacist.

Calcium carbonate

This is commonly included in OTC formulations. It acts quickly, has a prolonged action and is a potent neutralizer of acid. It can cause acid rebound and, if taken over long periods at high doses, can cause hypercalcaemia and so should not be recommended for long-term use. *Calcium carbonate* and *sodium bicarbonate* can, if taken in large quantities with a high intake of milk, result in the milk–alkali syndrome. This involves hypercalcaemia, metabolic alkalosis and renal insufficiency; its symptoms are nausea, vomiting, anorexia, headache and mental confusion.

Dimethicone

Dimethicone is sometimes added to antacid formulations for its defoaming properties. Theoretically, it reduces surface tension and allows easier elimination of gas from the gut by passing flatus or eructation (belching).

Interactions with antacids

Because they raise the gastric pH, antacids can interfere with enteric coatings on tablets which are intended to release their contents further along the GI tract. The consequences of this may be that release of the drug is unpredictable; adverse effects may occur if the drug is in contact with the stomach. Alternatively, enteric coatings are sometimes used to protect a drug which may be inactivated by the low pH in the stomach, so concurrent administration of antacids may result in such inactivation.

Sucralfate works best in an acid medium, so concurrent administration with antacids should be avoided. Excretion of *flecainide, mexiletine* and *quinidine* may be reduced and plasma levels increased if the urine is alkaline and antacids may increase urinary pH. Antacids may reduce the absorption of tetracyclines, *azithromycin, itraconazole, ketoconazole, penicillamine, chlorpromazine, diflunisal, dipyridamole, ciprofloxacin, norfloxacin, ofloxacin, piyampicillin* and *rifampicin. Sodium bicarbonate* may increase the excretion of *lithium* and lower the plasma level, so that a reduction in *lithium's* therapeutic effect may occur. Antacids containing *sodium bicarbonate* should not therefore be recommended for any patient on *lithium* therapy.

The changes in pH which occur after antacid administration can result in a decrease in iron absorption if *iron* is taken at the same time. The effect is caused by the formation of insoluble iron salts due to the changed pH. Taking *iron* and antacids at different times should prevent the problem.

Interactions:

azithromycin
chlorpromazine
ciprofloxacin, norfloxacin, ofloxacin
diflunisal
dipyridamole
enteric coated tablets
ketoconazole, itraconazole
lithium
penicillamine
pivampicillin
quinidine
rifampicin
sucralfate
tetracyclines.

Cimetidine, famotidine and ranitidine

These H_2 antagonists have been deregulated from prescription only status for the short-term treatment of dyspepsia and heartburn (see also p. 69). *Cimetidine* affects the cytochrome P450 enzyme system in the liver and therefore produces a range of drug interactions (see p. 70); *famotidine* and *ranitidine* do not affect the cytochrome P450 system. Treatment with these drugs is limited to a maximum of 2 weeks.

Discussing the use of H_2 antagonists with local family doctors would be valuable. Perhaps agreeing general guidelines or a protocol for their use could be a feature of the discussion.

Indigestion in practice

Case 1

Mrs Johnson, an elderly woman, complains of 'indigestion' and 'an upset stomach'. On questioning, you find out she has had the problem for a few days; the pain is epigastric and does not seem to be related to food. She has been feeling slightly nauseated. You ask about her diet; she has not changed her diet recently and has not been 'overdoing it'. She tells you that she is taking four lots of tablets; for her heart, her 'waterworks' and some new ones for her bad hip (*indomethacin* 25 mg three times a day). She has been taking them after meals, as advised and has not tried any medicines yet to treat her symptoms. Before the *indomethacin*, she was taking *paracetamol* for the pain. She normally uses *paracetamol* as a general painkiller at home—she tells you that she cannot take *aspirin* because it upsets her stomach.

The pharmacist's view

It sounds as though this woman is suffering GI symptoms as a result of her NSAID. Such effects are more common in elderly patients. She has been taking the medicine after food, which should have minimized any GI effects and the best course of action would be to refer her back to the doctor. It would be worth reminding Mrs Johnson always to check before using home painkillers in addition to those prescribed by the doctor in future. She might otherwise inadvertently duplicate *paracetamol* doses.

The doctor's view

Referral back to her doctor is the correct course of action. Almost certainly her symptoms have been caused by the *indomethacin*. She should be advised to stop it and see whether or not her symptoms improve. A short course of an antacid may speed up resolution. If an ulcer is suspected, treatment with an H_2 antagonist may be started.

Control of her primary symptom (hip pain) will then be a problem. NSAIDs should be avoided, especially if her pain is due to osteoarthritis. It may be possible to change the *paracetamol* to a compound preparation containing *paracetamol* and *codeine* or *dihydrocodeine*.

Rarely, if an NSAID is necessary to control the pain and there is a documented history of peptic ulceration, an NSAID may be given concomitantly with *misoprostol*. *Misoprostol* is a prostaglandin analogue which protects the gastric mucosa and may limit damage from NSAIDs. Failure to control hip pain due to osteoarthritis may require referral to an orthopaedic surgeon to consider a hip replacement.

Case 2

Ken Jones is a local milkman in his early fifties and he comes in to ask your advice about his stomach trouble. He tells you that he has been having the problem for a couple of months but it seems to have got worse. The pain is in his stomach, quite high up; he had similar pain a few months ago, but it got better and has now come back again. The pain seems to get better after a meal; sometimes it wakes him during the night. He has been taking Rennies to treat his symptoms; they did the trick, but don't seem to be working now, even though he takes a lot of them and he has also been taking some Aludrox Liquid. He is not taking any other medicines.

The pharmacist's view

Mr Jones has a history of epigastric pain, which remitted and has now returned. At one stage his symptoms responded to an antacid but they no longer do so, despite his increasing the dose. This long history, the worsening symptoms and the failure of medication warrants referral to the doctor.

The doctor's view

It would be sensible to recommend referral to his doctor as the information obtained so far does not permit diagnosis. It is possible that Mr Jones has a stomach ulcer, acid reflux or even a stomach cancer, but further information is required. An appropriate examination and investigation will be necessary.

The doctor would need to listen carefully first by asking open questions and by asking then more direct, closed questions to find out more information, for example: how does the pain affect him? What is the nature of the pain (burning, sharp, dull, tight, constricting)? Does it radiate (to back or chest, down arms, up to neck/mouth)? Are there any associated symptoms (nausea, difficulty in swallowing, loss of appetite, weight loss, shortness of breath? Are there any other problems (constipation, flatulence)? What are the aggravating/relieving factors? How is his general health? What is his diet like? How are things going for him generally (personally/professionally)? Does he smoke? How much alcohol does he drink? What does he think might be wrong with him? What are his expectations for treatment/management?

Further investigation may be necessary to clarify the diagnosis. This could be achieved by an endoscopy or a barium swallow/meal. The former is the more accurate method and allows for a biopsy to be taken. A biopsy is helpful in determining whether an ulcer is benign or malignant and for identification of the presence of a bacterium called *Helicobacter pylori*. There is increasing support for the causative role of *H. pylori* in peptic ulcers. This bacterium is present in nearly all cases of duodenal ulceration and over 80% of those with gastric ulceration. Treatment to eradicate *H. pylori* appears to be very successful in reducing the chances of future ulcer recurrence. This is particularly significant as the natural history is one of repeated relapse. The most effective treatment to eradicate *H. pylori* is 'triple therapy' and is detailed in the *British National Formulary*.

Nausea and vomiting

Nausea and vomiting are symptoms which have many possible causes. From the pharmacist's point of view, while there are treatments available to prevent nausea and vomiting, there is no effective over-the-counter (OTC) treatment once vomiting is established. For that reason, this section will deal briefly with some of the causes of these symptoms and then go on in the next section to consider the prevention of motion sickness, where the pharmacist can recommend effective treatments to help prevent the problem.

<table>
<tr><td>What you need to know</td></tr>
<tr><td>Age
  Infant, child, adult, elderly
Pregnancy
Duration
Symptoms
  Has vomiting started?
  Abdominal pain
  Diarrhoea
  Constipation
  Fever
Alcohol intake
Medication
  Prescribed
  OTC
Previous history
  Dizziness/vertigo</td></tr>
</table>

Significance of questions and answers

Age

The very young and the elderly are most at risk from dehydration as a result of vomiting. Vomiting of milk in infants less than a year old may be due to infection or feeding problems or, rarely, to an obstruction such as pyloric stenosis. In the latter there is thickening of the muscular wall around the outlet of the stomach which causes a blockage. It typically occurs in the first few weeks of life in a first-born male. The vomiting is frequently projectile in that the vomit is forcibly expelled a considerable distance. The condition can be cured by a simple operation. The pharmacist must distinguish, by questioning, between vomiting (the forced expulsion of gastric contents through the mouth) and regurgitation (where food is effortlessly brought up from the throat and stomach). Regurgitation sometimes occurs in babies, where it is known as 'posseting' and is a normal occurrence; and also in adults, where it is associated with oesophageal disease and hence difficulty in swallowing (see p. 67). Nausea is associated with vomiting but not regurgitation and this can be employed as a distinguishing feature during questioning.

Pregnancy

Nausea and vomiting are very common in pregnancy, usually beginning after the first missed period and occurring early in the morning. Pregnancy should be considered as a possible cause of nausea and vomiting in any woman of child-bearing age who presents at the pharmacy complaining of nausea and vomiting. Nausea and vomiting are more common in the first pregnancy than in subsequent ones.

Duration

Generally, adults should be referred to the doctor if vomiting has been present for longer than 2 days. Infants and children under 2 years of age are referred whatever the duration because of the risks from dehydration. Anyone presenting with chronic vomiting should be referred to the doctor since such symptoms may indicate the presence of a peptic ulcer or gastric carcinoma.

Symptoms

An acute infection (gastroenteritis) is often responsible for vomiting and, in these cases, diarrhoea (see p. 103) may also be present. Careful questioning about food intake during the previous 2 days may give a clue as to the cause. In young children, the rotavirus is the most common cause of gastroenteritis, which is highly infectious and so it is not unusual for more than one child in the family to be affected. In such situations there are usually associated cold symptoms.

The vomiting of blood may indicate serious disease and is an indication for referral, since it may be caused by haemorrhage from a peptic ulcer or gastric carcinoma. Sometimes the trauma of vomiting can cause a small bleed, due to a tear in the gut lining. Vomit with a faecal smell means that the gastrointestinal (GI) tract may be obstructed and requires urgent referral.

Nausea and vomiting may be associated with a migraine (see p. 180).

Alcohol intake

People who drink large quantities of alcohol may vomit, often in the morning. This may be due to occasional binge drinking or to chronic ingestion of alcohol. Alcoholic patients often feel nauseous and retch in the mornings. The questioning of patients about their intake of alcohol is a sensitive area and should be approached with tact. Asking about smoking habits might be a good way of introducing other social habits.

Medication

Prescribed and OTC medicines may make patients feel sick and it is therefore important to determine which medicines the patient is currently taking. *Aspirin* and non-steroidal anti-inflammatory drugs (NSAIDs) are common causes. Some antibiotics may cause nausea and vomiting, for example, *doxycyline*. Oestrogens, steroids and narcotic analgesics may also produce these symptoms. Symptoms can sometimes be improved by taking the medication with food, but if they continue the patient should see the doctor. *Digoxin* toxicity may show itself by producing nausea and vomiting and such symptoms in a patient who is taking *digoxin*, especially an elderly person, should prompt immediate referral where questioning has not produced an apparent cause for the symptoms. Vomiting, with loss of fluids and possible electrolyte imbalances, may cause problems in elderly people taking *digoxin* and diuretics.

Previous history

Any history which suggests chronic nausea and vomiting would indicate referral. Any history of dizziness or vertigo should be noted, as it may point to inner ear disease as a cause of the nausea.

Management

Patients who are vomiting should be referred to the doctor, who will be able to prescribe an anti-emetic if needed. The pharmacist can initiate rehydration therapy in the meantime.

Motion sickness and its prevention

Motion sickness is thought to be caused by a conflict of messages to the brain, where the vomiting centre receives information from the eyes, the gastrointestinal (GI) tract and the vestibular system in the ear. Symptoms of motion sickness include nausea and sometimes vomiting, pallor and cold sweats. Parents commonly seek advice about how to prevent motion sickness in children, in whom the problem is most common. Any form of travel can produce symptoms, including air, sea and road. Effective prophylactic treatments are available over the counter (OTC) and can be selected to match the patient's needs.

What you need to know

Age
    Infant, child, adult
Previous history
Mode of travel
    Car, bus, air, ferry, etc.
Length of journey
Medication

Significance of questions and answers

Age

Motion sickness is common in young children. Babies and very young children up to 2 years old seem to only rarely suffer from the problem and therefore do not usually require treatment. The incidence of motion sickness seems to greatly reduce with age, although some adults still experience symptoms. The minimum age at which products designed to prevent motion sickness can be given varies, so for a family with several children careful product selection can provide one medicine to treat all cases.

Previous history

The pharmacist should ascertain which members of the family have previously experienced motion sickness and for whom treatment will be needed.

Mode of travel/length of journey

Details of the journey to be undertaken are useful. The estimated length of time to be spent travelling will help the pharmacist in the selection of prophylactic treatment, since the length of action of available drugs varies.

Once vomiting starts there is little that can be done, so any medicine recommended by the pharmacist must be taken in good time before the journey if it is to be effective. The fact that it is important that the symptoms are prevented before they can gain a hold should be emphasized to the parents. If it is a long journey it may be necessary to repeat the dose while travelling and the recommended dosage interval should be stressed.

The pharmacist can also offer useful general advice about reducing motion sickness according to the method of transport to be used. For example, children are less likely to feel or be sick if they can see out of the car, so appropriate seats can be used to elevate the seating position of small children. This seems to be effective in practice and is thought to be because it allows the child to see relatively still objects outside the car. This ability to focus on such objects may help to settle the brain's receipt of conflicting messages.

For any method of travel, children are less likely to experience symptoms if they are kept occupied by playing games as they are therefore concentrating on something else. However, again, it seems that looking outside at still objects remains helpful and that a simple game, for example, 'I Spy', is better than reading in this respect. In fact for many travel sickness sufferers reading exacerbates feeling of nausea.

Medication

In addition to checking any prescription or OTC medicines currently being taken, the pharmacist should also enquire about any treatments used in the past for motion sickness and their level of success or failure.

Management

Prophylactic treatments for motion sickness which can be bought OTC are effective and there is usually no need to refer patients to the doctor.

Anticholinergic activity is thought to prevent motion sickness and forms the basis of treatment by anticholinergic agents (e.g. *hyoscine*) and antihistamines, which have anticholinergic actions (e.g. *cinnarizine, promethazine*).

Antihistamines

These include *cinnarizine, meclozine, dimenhydrinate* and *promethazine*.

Anticholinergic effects are thought to be responsible for the effectiveness of antihistamines in the prophylaxis of motion sickness. All have the potential to cause drowsiness and *promethazine* appears to be the most sedative. *Meclozine* and *pronethazine theoclate* have long durations of action and are useful for long journeys since they only need to be taken once daily. *Cinnarizine* and *promethazine theoclate* are not recommended for children younger than 5 years of age, whereas *meclozine* can be given to those over 2 years of age. The manufacturers of products containing these drugs advise that they are best avoided during pregnancy.

Anticholinergic agents

The only anticholinergic used widely in the prevention of motion sickness is *hyoscine hydrobromide,* which can be given to children over 3 years old. Anticholinergic drugs can cause drowsiness, blurred vision, dry mouth, constipation and urinary retention as side effects, although they are probably unlikely to do so at the doses used in OTC formulations for motion sickness. Children could be given sweets to suck to counteract any drying of the mouth.

Hyoscine has a short duration of action (from 1 to 3 hours). It is therefore suitable for shorter journeys and should be given 20 minutes before the start of the journey. Anticholinergic drugs and antihistamines with anticholinergic effects are best avoided in patients with prostatic hypertrophy because of the possibility of urinary retention and in glaucoma because the intra-ocular pressure might be increased.

Pharmacists should remember that side effects from anticholinergic agents are additive and may be increased in patients already taking drugs with anticholinergic effects, such as *amantidine*, tricyclic antidepressants (e.g. *amitriptyline*), butyrophenones (e.g. *haloperidol*) and phenothiazines (e.g. *chlorpromazine*). It is therefore important for the pharmacist to determine the identity of any medicines currently being taken by the patient. Table 1 summarizes recommended doses and length of action for the treatments discussed.

Alternative approaches to motion sickness

Ginger

Some years ago it was found that ginger powder (*Zingiber officinale*) could effectively reduce motion sickness. No mechanism of action has been identified but it has been suggested that ginger acts on the GI tract itself rather than on the vomiting centre in the brain or on the vestibular system. No official dosage level has been suggested but several proprietary products containing ginger are available. Ginger would be worth trying for a driver who suffered from motion sickness, since it does not cause

Table 1 Treatments for motion sickness.

Ingredient	Minimum age for use (years)	Children's dose	Adult dose	Timing of 1st dose in relation to journey	Recommended dose interval (hours)
Cinnarizine	5	15 mg	30 mg	2 hours before	8
Dimenhydrinate	1	1–6 years: 12.5–25 mg 7–12 years: 25–50 mg	50–100 mg	30 minutes before	8–12
Hyoscine hydrobromide	3	3–4 years: 75 μg 4–7 years: 150 μg 7–12 years: 150–300 μg	300 μg	20 minutes before	6
Meclozine	2	2–12 years: 12.5 mg	25 mg	Previous evening or 1 hour before	24
Promethazine theoclate	5	5–10 years: 12.5 mg Over 10 years: 25 mg	25 mg	Previous evening or 1 hour before	24

drowsiness, and might be worth considering for use in pregnant women, for whom other anti-emetics such as anticholinergics and antihistamines are not recommended.

Acupressure wrist bands

Following their apparently successful use on board naval ships to reduce motion sickness, elasticated wrist bands which apply pressure to a defined point on the inside of the wrists are now readily available. As yet there is no consistent evidence from clinical trials of the effectiveness of this method but research is continuing. Such wrist bands might be worth trying for drivers or pregnant women.

Constipation

Constipation is a condition which is difficult to define and is often self-diagnosed by patients. Generally it is characterized by the passage of hard, dry stools less frequently than the person's normal pattern. It is important for the pharmacist to find out what the patient means by 'constipation', and to establish what (if any) change in bowel habit has occurred and over what period of time.

What you need to know

Details of bowel habit
    Frequency and nature of bowel actions now
    When was the last bowel movement?
    What is the usual bowel habit?
    When did the problem start?
    Is there a previous history?
Associated symptoms
    Abdominal pain/discomfort/bloating/distension
    Nausea and vomiting
    Blood in the stool
Diet
    Any recent change in diet?
    Is the usual diet rich in fibre?
Medication
    Present medication
    Any recent change in medication
    Previous use of laxatives

Significance of questions and answers

Details of bowel habit

Many people believe that a daily bowel movement is necessary for good health and laxatives are often taken and abused as a result. In fact, the 'normal' range may vary from three movements in 1 day to three in 1 week. Therefore an important health education role for the pharmacist is in reassuring patients that their frequency of bowel movement is 'normal'. Patients who are constipated will usually complain of hard stools which are difficult to pass and less frequent than usual.

The determination of any change in bowel habit is essential, particularly any prolonged change. A sudden change which has lasted for 2 weeks or longer would be an indication for referral.

Associated symptoms

Constipation is often associated with abdominal discomfort, bloating and nausea. In some cases constipation can be so severe as to obstruct the bowel. This obstruction or blockage usually becomes evident by causing colicky abdominal pain, abdominal distension and vomiting. When symptoms suggestive of obstruction are present, urgent referral is necessary as hospital admission is the usual course of action. Constipation is only one of many possible causes of obstruction. Other causes such as bowel tumours or twisted bowels (volvulus) require urgent surgical intervention.

Blood in the stool

The presence of blood in the stool can be associated with constipation and although alarming is not necessarily serious. In such situations blood may arise from piles (haemorrhoids) or a small crack in the skin on the edge of the anus (anal fissure). Both these conditions are thought to be caused by a diet low in fibre which tends to produce constipation. The bleeding is characteristically noted on toilet paper after defaecation. The bright red blood may be present on the surface of the motion (not mixed in with the stool) and splashed around the toilet pan. If piles are present there is often discomfort on defaecation. The piles may drop down (prolapse) and protrude through the anus. A fissure tends to cause less bleeding but much more severe pain on defaecation. Medical referral is usually advisable as there are other more serious causes of bloody stools, especially where the blood is mixed in with the motion.

Bowel cancer

Bowel cancer may also present with a persisting change in bowel habit. This condition kills more than 20 000 people each year in the UK. Early diagnosis and intervention can dramatically improve the prognosis. Bowel cancer is more common in those over 50 years old but can, rarely, also occur in younger age groups.

Diet

Insufficient dietary fibre is a common cause of constipation. An impression of the fibre content of the diet can be gained by asking what would normally be eaten during a day, looking particularly for the presence of wholemeal cereals, bread, fresh fruit and vegetables. Changes in diet and lifestyle, for example, following a job change, loss of work, retirement, or travel may result in constipation. An inadequate intake of food and fluids, for example, in someone who has been ill, may be responsible.

Medication

One or more laxatives may already have been taken in an attempt to treat the symptoms. Failure of such medication may indicate that referral to the doctor is the best option. Previous history of the use of laxatives is relevant. Continuous use, especially of stimulant laxatives, can result in a vicious circle where the contents of the gut are expelled, causing a subsequent cessation of bowel actions for 1 or 2 days. This then leads to the false conclusion that constipation has recurred and more laxatives are taken, and so on.

Chronic overuse of stimulant laxatives can result in loss of muscular activity in the bowel wall (an atonic colon) and thus further constipation.

Many drugs can induce constipation; some examples are listed in Table 2. The details of prescribed and over-the-counter (OTC) medication being taken should be established.

When to refer
Change in bowel habit of 2 weeks or longer
Presence of abdominal pain, vomiting, bloating
Blood in stools
Prescribed medication suspected of causing symptoms
Failure of OTC medication

Table 2 Drugs which may cause constipation.

Analgesics and opiates	*Dihydrocodeine, codeine*
Antacids	*Aluminium salts*
Anticholinergics	*Hyoscine*
Anticonvulsants	*Phenytoin*
Antidepressants	*Amitriptyline*
Antihistamines	*Chlorpheniramine, promethazine*
Antihypertensives	*Clonidine, prazosin, methyldopa*
Anti-Parkinson agents	*Levodopa*
Beta blockers	*Propranolol*
Diuretics	*Bendrofluazide*
Iron	
Laxative abuse	
Monoamine oxidase inhibitors	*Phenelzine*
Psychotropics	*Chlorpromazine*

Treatment timescale

If 1 week's use of treatment does not produce relief of symptoms the patient should see the doctor. If the pharmacist feels that it is only necessary to give dietary advice, then it would be reasonable to leave it for about 2 weeks to see if the symptoms settle.

Management

Constipation which is not caused by serious pathology will usually respond to simple measures which can be recommended by the pharmacist: increasing the amount of dietary fibre; maintaining fluid consumption; and taking regular exercise. In the short term, a laxative may be recommended to ease the immediate problem.

Stimulant laxatives (e.g. *senna, bisacodyl*)

These work by increasing peristalsis. All stimulant laxatives can produce griping/cramping pains. It is advisable to start at the lower end of the recommended dosage range, increasing the dose if needed. The intensity of the laxative effect is related to the dose taken. Stimulant laxatives work within 6–12 hours when taken orally. They should be used for a maximum of 1 week. *Bisacodyl* tablets are enteric coated and should be swallowed whole because bisacodyl is irritant to the stomach. If it is given as a suppository, the effect usually occurs within an hour and sometimes as soon as 15 minutes after insertion.

Docusate sodium appears to have both stimulant and stool-softening effects and acts within 1–2 days.

The use of *senna pods* and *cascara* which is non-standardized should be discouraged because the dose, and therefore action, are unpredictable *Phenolphthalein* should be avoided altogether because it is absorbed and can produce unpleasant side effects. The absorbed *phenolphthalein* is excreted with bile back into the GI tract (an enterohepatic cycle) where a laxative effect will be exerted. The cycle continues and the laxative action of *phenolphthalein* can last for 3–4 days. Adverse effects including albuminuria, rashes and haemoglobinuria may also occur.

Castor oil is a traditional remedy for constipation which is no longer recommended. Evacuation of the bowel occurs within 2–6 hours. Castor oil works best if taken on an empty stomach but it has an unpleasant taste and can cause griping pains. Its use is best avoided since there are better preparations available.

Bulk laxatives (e.g. *ispaghula, methylcellulose, sterculia*)

These are the laxatives which most closely copy the normal physiological mechanisms involved in bowel evacuation and are considered by many to be the laxatives of choice. Such agents are especially useful where patients cannot or will not increase their intake of dietary fibre. Bulk laxatives work by swelling in the gut and increasing faecal mass so that peristalsis is stimulated. The laxative effect can take several days to develop.

The sodium content of bulk laxatives (as *sodium bicarbonate*) should be considered in those requiring a restricted sodium intake.

When recommending the use of a bulk laxative, the pharmacist should advise that an increase in fluid intake will be necessary. In the form of granules or powder, the preparation should be mixed with a full glass of liquid (e.g. fruit juice or water) before taking. Fruit juice can mask the bland taste of the preparation. Intestinal obstruction may result from inadequate fluid intake in patients taking bulk laxatives, particularly those whose gut is not functioning properly as a result of abuse of stimulant laxatives.

Osmotic laxatives (e.g. *lactulose, Epsom salts, Glauber's salts*)

Epsom salts (magnesium sulphate) and *Glauber's salts (sodium sulphate)* act by drawing water into the gut; the increased pressure which results increases intestinal motility. A dose of either salt usually produces a bowel movement within a few hours. *Glauber's salts* should be avoided in those whose sodium intake needs to be restricted. Occasional use of *Epsom* or *Glauber's salts* can be useful where a rapid evacuation of the bowel is needed, but they are unsuitable for long-term use because their repeated use can lead to dehydration. *Lactulose* works by maintaining the volume of fluid in the bowel. It may take 1–2 days to work. *Lactitol* is chemically related to *lactulose* and is available as sachets. The contents of the sachet are taken sprinkled on food or with liquid. One or two glasses of fluid should be taken with the daily dose.

Glycerin suppositories have both osmotic and irritant effects and usually act within an hour. They may cause rectal discomfort. Moistening the suppository before use will make insertion easier.

Lubricant laxatives (e.g. *liquid paraffin*)

Liquid paraffin works by coating and softening the faeces; it prevents further absorption of water in the colon. Long-term use can results in impaired absorption of fat-soluble vitamins (A, D, E, K). Leakage of *liquid paraffin* through the anal sphincter may occur, causing embarassment and unpleasantness. If *liquid paraffin* is inadvertently inhaled into the lungs a lipid pneumonia can develop. Inhalation could occur during vomiting or if acid reflux (regurgitation) is present. The unpleasant and dangerous effects of *liquid paraffin* have led to restrictions in the UK on the pack size which can be sold. Pharmacists have an important role in discouraging the use of *liquid paraffin*, which has little valid therapeutic use.

Constipation in children

Parents sometimes ask for laxatives for use by children. Fixed ideas about 'regular' bowel habits are often responsible for such requests. Numerous factors can cause constipation in children, including a change in diet and emotional causes. Simple advice about sufficient dietary fibre may be all that is needed.

If the problem is of recent origin and there are no significant associated signs, a single *glycerin suppository* together with dietary advice may be appropriate. Referral to the doctor would be best if these measures are unsuccessful.

Constipation in pregnancy

Constipation commonly occurs during pregnancy; hormonal changes are responsible and it has been estimated that one in three pregnant women suffers from constipation. Dietary advice concerning the intake of plenty of high-fibre foods and fluids can help. *Oral iron*, often prescribed for pregnant women, may contribute to the problem.

Stimulant laxatives are best avoided during pregnancy; bulk-forming laxatives are preferable, although they may cause some abdominal discomfort to women when used late in pregnancy.

Constipation in the elderly

Constipation is a common problem in elderly patients for several reasons: elderly patients are less likely to be physically active; they often have poor natural teeth or false teeth and so may avoid high-fibre foods which are more difficult to chew; multi-drug regimens are more likely in elderly patients, who may therefore suffer from drug-induced constipation; fixed ideas about what constitutes a 'normal' bowel habit are common in older patients. If a bulk laxative is to be recommended for an elderly patient, it is of great importance that the pharmacist gives advice about maintaining fluid intake to prevent the possible development of intestinal obstruction.

Laxative abuse

Two groups of patients are likely to abuse laxatives: those with chronic constipation who get into a vicious circle by using stimulant laxatives (see p. 94), which eventually results in damage to the nerve plexus in the colon; and those who take laxatives in the belief that they will control weight, for example, those who are dieting or, more seriously, women with eating disorders (anorexia nervosa or bulimia), who take very large quantities of laxatives. The pharmacist is in a position to monitor purchases of laxative products and counsel patients as appropriate. Any patient who is ingesting large amounts of laxative agents should be referred to the doctor.

Constipation in practice

Case 1

Mr Johnson is a middle-aged man who occasionally visits your pharmacy. Today he complains of constipation, which he has had for several weeks. He has been having a bowel movement every few days; normally they are every day or every other day. His motions are hard and painful to pass. He has not tried any medicines as he thought the problem would go of its own accord. He has never had problems with constipation in the past. He has been taking *atenolol* tablets 50 mg once a day, for over a year. He does not have any other symptoms, except a slight feeling of abdominal discomfort. You ask him about his diet; he tells you that since he was made redundant from his job at a local factory 3 months ago he has tended to eat less than usual; his dietary intake sounds as if it is low in fibre. He tells you that he has been applying for jobs, with no success so far. He says he feels really 'down' and is starting to think that he may never get another job.

The pharmacist's view

Mr Johnson's symptoms are almost certainly due to the change in his lifestyle and eating pattern. Now he is not working he is likely to be less physically active and his eating pattern has probably changed. From what he has said, it sounds as if he is becoming depressed because of his lack of success in finding work. Constipation seems to be associated with depression, separately from the constipating effect of some anti-depressant drugs.

It would be worth asking Mr Johnson if he is sleeping well (signs of clinical depression include disturbed sleep; either difficulty in getting to sleep or waking early and not being able to get back to sleep). Weight can change either way in depression. Some patients eat for comfort, while others find their appetite is reduced. Depending on his response you might consider whether referral to his doctor is needed.

To address the dietary problems, he could be advised to start the day with a wholemeal cereal and to eat at least four slices of wholemeal bread each day. Baked beans are a cheap, good source of fibre. Fresh vegetables are also fibre-rich. It would be important to stress that fluid intake should also be increased. A high-fibre diet means patients should increase their fibre intake until they pass one large, soft stool each day;

the amount of fibre needed to produce this effect will vary markedly between patients. The introduction of dietary fibre should be gradual; too rapid an increase can cause griping and wind.

To provide relief from the discomfort, a suppository of *glycerin* or *bisacodyl* could be recommended to produce a bowel evacuation quickly; in the longer term, dietary changes provide the key. He should see the doctor if the suppository does not produce an effect; if it works but the dietary changes have not been effective after 2 weeks, he should go to his doctor. Mr Johnson's medication is unlikely to be responsible for his constipation because, although beta blockers can sometimes cause constipation, he has been taking the drug for over a year with no previous problems.

The doctor's view

The advice given by the pharmacist is sensible. It is likely that Mr Johnson's physical and mental health have been affected by the impact of a significant change in his life. The loss of his job and the uncertainty of future employment is a major and continuing source of stress. The fact that the pharmacist has taken time to check out how he has been affected will in itself be therapeutic. It also gives the pharmacist the opportunity to refer to the doctor if necessary. Many people are reluctant to take such problems to their doctor but a recommendation from the pharmacist might make the process easier. Hopefully the advice given for constipation will at least improve one aspect of his life. If the constipation does not resolve within 2 weeks Mr Johnson should see his doctor.

Case 2

Your counter assistant asks if you will have a word with a young woman who is in the shop. She was recognized by your assistant as a regular purchaser of stimulant laxatives. You explain to the woman that you will need to ask a few questions because regular use of laxatives may mean an underlying problem which is not improving. In answer to your questions she tells you that she diets almost constantly and always suffers from constipation. Her weight appears to be within the range for her height. You show her your pharmacy's body mass index chart and work out with her where she is on the chart, which confirms your initial feeling. However, she is reluctant to accept your advice, saying that she definitely needs to lose some more weight. You ask about her diets and she tells you that she has tried all sorts of approaches, most of which involve eating very little.

The pharmacist's view

Unfortunately, this sort of story is all too common in community pharmacy, with many women who seek to achieve weight below the recommended range. The pharmacist can explain that constipation often occurs during dieting simply because insufficient bulk and fibre is being eaten to allow the gut to work normally. Perhaps the pharmacist might suggest that she joins a local group, either Weight Watchers or a self-help group (the local health promotion unit will know what is available). Despite the pharmacist's advice, many customers will still wish to purchase laxatives and the pharmacist will need to consider how to handle refusal of sales. Offering stimulant laxatives for sale by self-selection can only exacerbate the problems and make it more difficult to monitor sales and refuse them when necessary.

The doctor's view

This is obviously a difficult problem for the pharmacist. It is inappropriate for the young woman to continue taking laxatives and she could benefit from counselling. However, a challenge from the pharmacist could result in her simply buying the laxatives elsewhere. If, as is likely, she has an eating disorder she may have very low self-esteem and be denying her problem. Both of these factors make it more difficult for the pharmacist to intervene most effectively. An ideal outcome would be appropriate referral, which would depend on local resources but which might initially be to the doctor.

If she is seen by the doctor, a gentle and sympathetic approach is necessary. The most important thing is to give her full opportunity to say what she thinks about the problem, how it makes her feel, and how it affects her life. Establishing a supportive relationship with resultant trust between patient and doctor is the major aim of the initial consultation. Once this has been achieve further therapeutic opportunities can be discussed and decided on together.

Case 3

Mrs McConnell is a woman aged about 45 whom you know well. She is a regular customer, who has often sought your advice about her children's health. She wants you to recommend something for constipation, which she has had for about 3 weeks. She generally has a bowel movement every day and has only passed a motion twice during the last 10 days; she has not felt or been sick and has no other symptoms, but says she feels as though she wants to go to the toilet, but cannot. Her last two motions were difficult and painful to pass. She has tried some laxatives which seemed to work but the problem has come back. She tells you that she has been feeling 'down in the dumps' recently and that the doctor gave her some tablets to make her feel better. You remember dispensing a prescription for some *imipramine* tablets for her a few weeks ago and confirm this using your patient medication records. She is not taking any other medicines.

The pharmacist's view

This woman's constipation is likely to have been caused by her prescription medication; tricyclic antidepressants can cause constipation because of their anticholinergic side effects. The explanation is confirmed by the fact that this woman has tried a laxative, which worked, but then the constipation returned. Mrs McConnell should be encouraged to go back to her doctor and discuss the problem with him.

The doctor's view

Tricyclic antidepressant therapy is often complicated by constipation and a dry mouth. The constipation can often be prevented by anticipating the problem and giving dietary advice. If constipation is already a problem before starting tricyclics then it may be advisable to take a bulk laxative also. Referral back to the doctor is sensible in this situation. Mrs McConnell and her doctor can then decide whether or not to continue with antidepressants and how best to tackle the constipation. It may also provide an opportunity to explore her depression further and look at non-drug solutions, for example counselling.

Diarrhoea

Community pharmacists may be asked by patients to treat existing diarrhoea, or to offer advice on what course of action to take should diarrhoea occur, for example, to holidaymakers. Diarrhoea is defined as an increased frequency of bowel evacuation, with the passage of abnormally soft or watery faeces. The basis of treatment is electrolyte and fluid replacement; in addition, antidiarrhoeals are useful in adults and older children.

What you need to know

Age
   Infant, child, adult, elderly
Duration
Severity
Symptoms, associated symptoms
   Nausea/vomiting
   Fever
   Abdominal cramps
   Flatulence
   Other family members affected?
Previous history
Recent travel abroad?
Causative factors
Medication
   Medicines already tried
   Other medicines being taken

Significance of questions and answers

Age

Particular care is needed in the very young and the very old. Infants (younger than 1 year old) and elderly patients are especially at risk of becoming dehydrated.

Duration

Most cases of diarrhoea will be acute and self-limiting. Because of the dangers of dehydration it would be wise to refer infants with diarrhoea of longer than 1 day's duration to the doctor.

Severity

The degree of severity of diarrhoea is related to the nature and frequency of stools. Both these aspects are important, since misunderstandings can arise, especially in self-diagnosed complaints. Elderly patients who complain of diarrhoea may, in fact, be suffering from faecal impaction. They may pass liquid stools, but with only one or two bowel movements a day.

Symptoms

Acute diarrhoea is rapid in onset and produces watery stools which are passed frequently. Abdominal cramps, flatulence and weakness or malaise may also occur. Nausea and vomiting may be associated with diarrhoea, as may fever. The pharmacist should always ask about vomiting and fever in infants; both will increase the likelihood that severe dehydration will develop. Another important question to ask about diarrhoea in infants is whether the baby has been taking milk feeds and other drinks as normal. Reduced fluid intake predisposes to dehydration.

The pharmacist should question the patient about food intake and also about whether other family members or friends are suffering from the same symptoms, since acute diarrhoea is often infective in origin. Often there are localized minor outbreaks of gastroenteritis and the pharmacist may be asked several times for advice and treatment by different patients during a short period of time. Types of infective diarrhoea are discussed later in the chapter.

The presence of blood or mucus in the stools is an indication for referral. Diarrhoea with severe vomiting or with a high fever would also require medical advice.

Previous history

A previous history of diarrhoea or a prolonged change in bowel habit would warrant referral for further investigation and it is important that the pharmacist distinguishes between acute and chronic conditions. Chronic diarrhoea (of more than 3 weeks' duration) may be caused by bowel conditions such as Crohn's disease, irritable bowel syndrome (IBS) or ulcerative colitis and requires medical advice.

Recent travel abroad

Diarrhoea in a patient who has recently travelled abroad requires referral since it might be infective in origin.

Causes of diarrhoea

Infections

Most cases of diarrhoea are short lived, the bowel habit being normal before and after. In these situations the cause is likely to be infective (viral or bacterial).

Viral. Viruses are often responsible for gastroenteritis. In infants the virus causing such problems is often one which gains entry into the body via the respiratory tract (rotavirus). Associated symptoms are those of a cold and perhaps a cough. The infection starts abruptly and vomiting often precedes diarrhoea. The acute phase is usually over within 2–3 days, although diarrhoea may persist. Sometimes diarrhoea returns when milk feeds are reintroduced. This is because one of the milk digestive enzymes is temporarily inactivated. Milk therefore passes through the bowel undigested, causing diarrhoea. The health visitor or doctor would need to give further advice in such situations.

Whilst in the majority the infection is usually not too severe and is self-limiting, it should be remembered that rotavirus infection can cause death. This is most likely in those infants already malnourished and living in poor social circumstances who have not been breast fed.

Bacterial. These infections are the cause of food poisoning, which typically occurs when poultry is undercooked or contaminated food is reheated insufficiently. Two commonly seen types of infection are *Campylobacter* and *Salmonella*. In the latter, symptoms may arise 6–24 hours after ingestion of the infected food. There is an abrupt onset of frequent diarrhoea, occasionally with abdominal pain and vomiting. In the UK in recent years, *salmonella* has been linked to infected eggs, leading to a public health effort to ensure that eggs are thoroughly cooked before eating.

In *Campylobacter* infection there may be a longer incubation period (48–72 hours) and colicky abdominal pain is more common. Bloody diarrhoea may occur. The mainstay of treatment is fluid replacement. The infection is usually self-limiting and eliminated quickly from the bowel. Occasionally infection can persist in the bowel although symptoms have resolved (carrier state). This is of little consequence unless the carrier is the school cook or a restaurant chef. In such situations stool specimens have to be sent to the Public Health Laboratory until cleared.

Bacillus cereus has an incubation period of 1–6 hours and is usually associated with fried and boiled rice, especially if it has been kept warm or reheated.

Antibiotics are generally unnecessary and may cause additional problems due to side effects. They are occasionally needed in the most severe cases of salmonella infection when there may be signs of septicaemia, in cases of *Shigella* infection, or in severe campylobacter infection. *Ciprofloxacin* may be used in such circumstances.

Parasitic/protozoan. These infections are uncommon in western Europe but may occur in travellers returning from further afield. Examples include amoebic dysentery (giardiasis) and a worm infection, strongyloidiasis. Diagnosis is made by sending stool samples to the laboratory.

Chronic diarrhoea

Recurrent or persistent diarrhoea may be due to an irritable bowel or, more seriously, a bowel tumour, an inflammation of the bowel (e.g. ulcerative colitis or Crohn's disease), an inability to digest or absorb food (malabsorption; e.g. coeliac disease) or diverticular disease of the colon.

Irritable bowel syndrome (see p. 112). This non-serious but troublesome condition is one of the more common causes of recurrent bowel dysfunction in adolescents and young adults. The patient usually describes the frequent passage of small volumes of stool rather than true diarrhoea. The stools are typically variable in nature, often loose and semi-formed. They may be described as being like rabbit droppings or as pencil shaped. The frequency of bowel action is also variable as the diarrhoea may alternate with constipation. Often the bowels are open several times in the morning before the patient leaves for work. The condition is more likely to occur at times of stress, it may be associated with anxiety and occasionally it may be triggered by a bowel infection. Inadequate dietary fibre may also be of significance. It is possible that certain foods can irritate the bowel but this is difficult to prove.

There is no blood present within the motion in an irritable bowel. The presence of bloody diarrhoea may be as a result of an inflammation or tumour of the bowel. The latter is more likely with increasing age (from middle age onwards) and is likely to be associated with a prolonged change in bowel habit, with diarrhoea sometimes alternating with constipation.

Medication

Medicines already tried

The pharmacist should establish the identity of any medication which has already been taken to treat the symptoms in order to assess its appropriateness.

Other medicines being taken

Details of any other medication being taken (both over the counter (OTC)

Table 3 Some drugs which may cause diarrhoea.

Antacids: magnesium salts
Antibiotics
Antihypertensives: *guanethidine* (common); *methyldopa*; beta blockers
  (rare)
Digoxin (toxic levels)
Diuretics (e.g. *frusemide*)
Iron preparations
Laxatives
Misoprostol
Non-steroidal anti-inflammatory drugs

---

and prescribed) are also needed, as the diarrhoea may be drug-induced
(see Table 3). Over-the-counter medicines should be considered; commonly used medicines such as magnesium-containing antacids and iron
preparations are examples of medicines that may induce diarrhoea.
Laxative abuse should be considered as a possible cause.

When to refer

Diarrhoea of greater than 1 day's duration in children younger than 1 year
  old; 2 days in children under 3 years old and elderly patients; 3 days in
  older children and adults
Association with severe vomiting and fever
Suspected drug-induced reaction to prescribed medicine
History of change in bowel habit
Presence of blood or mucus in the stools

Treatment timescale

One day in children, otherwise 2 days.

Management

Oral rehydration therapy

The risk of dehydration from diarrhoea is greatest in babies and
rehydration therapy is considered to be the standard treatment for acute
diarrhoea in babies and young children. Oral rehydration sachets may
be used with antidiarrhoeals in older children and adults. Rehydration
may still be initiated even if referral to the doctor is advised. Sachets of
powder for reconstitution are available; these contain sodium as chloride
and bicarbonate, glucose and potassium. The absorption of sodium is
facilitated in the presence of glucose. A variety of flavours are available.

It is essential that appropriate advice is given by the pharmacist about how reconstitution should be performed. Patients should be reminded that only water should be used to make the solution (never fruit or fizzy drinks) and that boiled and cooled water should be used for children younger than 1 year old. Boiling water should not be used, as it would cause the liberation of carbon dioxide. The solution can be kept for 24 hours if stored in a refrigerator. Fizzy, sugary drinks should never be used to make rehydration fluids, they will produce a hyperosmolar solution which may exacerbate the problem. The sodium content of such drinks, as well as the glucose content, may be high.

Home-made salt and sugar solutions should not be recommended, since the accuracy of electrolyte content cannot be guaranteed and is essential, especially in infants, young children and elderly patients. Special measuring spoons are available; their correct use would produce a more acceptable solution, but their use should be reserved for the treatment of adults, where electrolyte concentration is less crucial.

Quantities

Parents sometimes ask how much rehydration fluid should be given to children. The following simple rules can be used for guidance; the amount of solution offered to the patient is based on the number of watery stools which are passed (Table 4).

Table 4 Amount of rehydration solution to be offered to patients.

Age	Quantity of solution (per watery stool)
Under 1 year	50 ml (quarter of a glass)
1–5 years	100 ml (half a glass)
6–12 years	200 ml (one glass)
Adults	400 ml (two glasses)

Other therapy

Loperamide

Loperamide is an effective antidiarrhoeal treatment for use in older children and adults. When recommending loperamide the pharmacist should remind patients to drink plenty of extra fluids. Oral rehydration sachets may be recommended. Loperamide may not be recommended for use in children under 12 years old.

Kaolin

This has been used as a traditional remedy for diarrhoea for many years. Its use was justified on the theoretical grounds that it would absorb water in the gastrointestinal (GI) tract and would adsorb toxins and bacteria onto its surface, thus removing them from the gut. The latter has not been shown to be true and the usefulness of the former is questionable. The use of *kaolin*-based preparations has largely been superseded by oral rehydration therapy, although patients continue to ask for various products containing *kaolin*.

Morphine

Morphine, in various forms, has been included in antidiarrhoeal remedies for many years. The theoretical basis for its inclusion is that *morphine*, together with other narcotic drugs such as *codeine*, is known to slow the action of the GI tract; indeed, constipation is a well-recognized side effect of such drugs. However, at the doses included in most OTC preparations it is unlikely that such an effect would be produced. *Kaolin and morphine mixture* remains a popular choice for some patients, despite the lack of evidence of its effectiveness.

Practical points

1 Patients with diarrhoea should be advised to drink plenty of clear, non-milky fluids, such as water and diluted squash.

2 Advice to eat no solid food for 24 hours may be appropriate. Breast or bottle feeding should be continued in infants. The severity and duration of diarrhoea are not affected by whether milk feeds are continued. A well-nourished child should be the aim, particularly where the infant is poorly nourished to begin with and where the withholding of milk feeds may be more detrimental than in a well-nourished infant, where temporary withdrawal is unimportant. Some doctors continue nevertheless to advise the discontinuation of milk, especially botttle, during the acute phase of infection.

3 Patients with diarrhoea might be best advised to avoid cow's milk, because during diarrhoea the enzyme in the gut which digests milk (lactase) is inactivated. A temporary lactose intolerance can therefore be produced, which makes the diarrhoea worse.

Diarrhoea in practice

Case 1

Mrs Robinson asks what you can recommend for diarrhoea. Her son David, aged 11, has diarrhoea and she is worried that her other two children, Natalie, aged 4 and Tom, aged just over 1 year, may also get it. David's diarrhoea started yesterday; he went to the toilet about five times and was sick once, but has not been sick since. He has griping pains, but is generally well and quite lively. For lunch yesterday he had pie and chips from the local takeaway during his lunchtime break at school. No one else in the family ate the same food. Mrs Robinson has not given him any medicine, but has some *kaolin and morphine mixture* at home and wants to know if David could take some of that and also the other children if necessary.

The pharmacist's view

It sounds as if David has a bout of acute diarrhoea, possibly caused by the food he ate yesterday lunchtime. He has vomited once, but now the diarrhoea is the problem. The child is otherwise well. He is 11 years old; the best plan would be to start oral rehydration with some proprietary sachets, with advice to his mother about how they should be reconstituted. *Kaolin and morphine mixture* should not be given to children under 12 years old, and in any case is not considered first-line treatment for diarrhoea. If either or both the other children get diarrhoea, they can also be given some rehydration solution. David should see the doctor the day after tomorrow if his condition has not improved.

The doctor's view

David's diarrhoea could well be due to food poisoning. Oral rehydration is the correct treatment. He should also be told not to eat anything for the next 24 hours or so until the diarrhoea has settled. If he wants to drink other fluids in addition to the electrolyte mixture, he should be told to avoid milk.

His symptoms should settle down over the next 24 hours. If they persist or he complains of worsening abdominal pain, particularly in the lower right side of the abdomen, his mother should contact the doctor. Rarely, an atypical acute appendicitis may present as a bowel infection.

Case 2

Mrs Jean Berry wants to stock up on some medicines before her family sets off on their first holiday abroad—they will be going to Spain next week. Mrs Berry tells you she has heard of people whose holidays have been ruined by holiday diarrhoea and she wants you to recommend a good treatment. On questioning, you find out that Mr and Mrs Berry and their two boys aged 10 and 14 will be going on the holiday.

The pharmacist's view

Holiday diarrhoea can be troublesome but can easily be dealt with. Mrs Berry could be advised to buy some *loperamide* capsules, which would be suitable treatment for herself, Mr Berry and their 14-year-old son. In addition, she should purchase some oral rehydration sachets for the younger son. The sachets could also be used by other family members.

The pharmacist could also give some valuable advice about avoidance of potential problems by the Berry family on their first foreign holiday. Fresh fruit should be peeled before eating and hot food should not be eaten other than in restaurants. Roadside snack stalls are best avoided. The question of the quality of the drinking water often crops up. Good advice to travellers would be to check with the tour company representative as to the advisability of drinking local water. If in doubt, bottled mineral water can be drunk; such water (the still variety) could also be used to reconstitute rehydration sachets. Ice in drinks may be best avoided, depending on the water supply.

Holiday diarrhoea is usually self-limiting, if it is still present after several days, medical advice should be sought. If the diarrhoea persists or is recurrent after returning home, the doctor should be seen. Finally, patients would be well advised to be wary of buying OTC medicines abroad. In some countries, a large range of drugs including oral steroids and antibiotics can be purchased over the counter. Each year, patients return to Britain with serious adverse effects following the use of oral *chloramphenicol*, for example, which has been prescribed or purchased.

The doctor's view

The pharmacist has covered all the important points. The most likely cause of diarrhoea would be contaminated food or water. The best treatment of acute diarrhoea is to stop eating and to drink bottled mineral water (with or without electrolyte reconstitution powders). It would be sensible to take an antidiarrhoeal such as *loperamide*.

Case 3

Mr Radcliffe is an elderly man who lives alone. Today, his home help asks what you can recommend for diarrhoea, from which Mr Radcliffe has been suffering for 3 days. He has been passing watery stools quite frequently and feels rather tired and weak. He has sent the home help because he dare not leave the house and go out of reach of the toilet. You check your patient medication records, which confirm your memory that he takes several different medicines; *digoxin*, *frusemide* and *paracetamol*. Last week you dispensed a prescription for a course of *amoxycillin*. The home help tells you that he has been eating his usual diet and there does not seem to be a link between food and his symptoms.

The pharmacist's view

Mr Radcliffe's diarrhoea may be due to the *amoxycillin*, which he started to take a few days ago. It would be best to call the patient's doctor to discuss the best course of action because Mr Radcliffe's other drug therapy means that fluid loss and dehydration may cause electrolyte imbalance and put him at further risk. The doctor may decide to stop the *amoxycillin*.

The doctor's view

It is likely that the *amoxycillin* has caused the diarrhoea. The most important consideration in management is to ensure adequate fluid and electrolyte replacement. This is particularly so as the elderly (and babies) are not as resilient to the effects of dehydration. In Mr Radcliffe's case things are further complicated by his other medication: *frusemide* and *digoxin*. He is not on any potassium supplement or a potassium-sparing diuretic. Although there may be good reason for this, diuretics such as *frusemide* can lower the plasma potassium level and make *digoxin* dangerously toxic. Unfortunately, potassium can also be lost in diarrhoea, further aggravating this problem. It is therefore reasonable to ask for the doctor to visit and assess.

There is also a small possibility that the diarrhoea could be due to pseudomembranous colitis (PMC) which is caused by a bacterium (*Clostridium difficile*) in the colon and typically occurs as a complication of antibiotic treatment. It is thought that antibiotics upset the normal bowel flora allowing *Clostridium difficile* to flourish. This is a rare condition which can be caused by most antibiotics but has been reported most often with *clindamycin, ampicillin, amoxycillin*, and the cephalosporins. The condition is more likely to occur in the elderly.

The diarrhoea of PMC can range from mild self-limiting symptoms to severe protracted or recurrent episodes and can sometimes be fatal. There is often a low-grade fever, and abdominal pain/cramps may occur. the symptoms usually begin within a week of starting antibiotic treatment but may start up to 6 weeks after a course of antibiotics. Where possible, antibiotics should be discontinued in cases of PMC. It is sometimes necessary to treat severe cases with *metronidazole* or *vancomycin*.

Irritable bowel syndrome

Irritable bowel syndrome (IBS) is defined as 'a functional bowel disorder in which abdominal pain is associated with defaecation or a change in bowel habit, with the additional features of disordered defaecation and abdominal distension'. Its cause is unknown. Irritable bowel syndrome is estimated to affect 20% of adults in the industrialized world, most of whom (up to three quarters) do not consult a doctor. More women with IBS consult a health professional than do men and the incidence of the condition appears to be higher in women. Debate has been fierce about whether IBS has a psychological cause because it is associated with anxiety or depression in many patients. However, differences in bowel sensitivity have been shown in IBS patients compared to those without IBS, although the full picture is not yet clear.

What you need to know

Age
   Child, adult
Symptoms
   Gastrointestinal
      Abdominal pain
      Abdominal distension/bloating
      Disturbed bowel habit; diarrhoea and/or constipation
      Nausea
   Other
      Urinary symptoms especially frequency
      Dyspareunia (pain during intercourse)
      Backache
      Fatigue
Duration
Previous history
Aggravating factors
   Stress; dietary (caffeine, sorbitol, fructose)
Medication

Significance of questions and answers

Age

Because of the difficulties in diagnosis of abdominal pain in children it is best to refer.

Irritable bowel syndrome often develops in young adult life. If an older person is presenting for the first time with no previous history of bowel problems a referral should be made.

Symptoms

Irritable bowel syndrome has three key symptoms:
abdominal pain (may ease following a bowel movement)
abdominal distension/bloating
disturbance of bowel habit.

Abdominal pain

The pain can occur anywhere in the abdomen. It is often central or left sided and can be severe. When pain occurs in the upper abdomen it can be confused with peptic ulcer or gall bladder pain. The site of pain can vary from person to person and even for an individual. Sometimes the pain comes on after eating and can be relieved by defaecation.

Bloating

A sensation of bloating is commonly reported. Sometimes it is so severe that clothes have to be loosened.

Bowel habit

Diarrhoea and constipation may occur; sometimes they alternate. A 'morning rush' is common, where the patient feels an urgent desire to defaecate several times after getting up in the morning and following breakfast, after which the bowel may settle. There may be a feeling of incomplete emptying after a bowel movement. The motion is often described as loose and semi-formed rather than watery. Sometimes it is like pellets or rabbit droppings, or pencil shaped. There may be mucus present but never blood.

Other symptoms

Nausea sometimes occurs, vomiting is less common.

Patients may also complain of apparently unrelated symptoms such as backache: feeling lethargic and tired. Urinary symptoms may be associated with IBS, for example, frequency, urgency and nocturia (the need to pass urine during the night). Some women report dyspareunia.

Duration

Patients may present when the first symptoms occur, or may describe a pattern of symptoms which has been going on for months or even years. If an older person is presenting for the first time referral is most appropriate.

Previous history

You need to know whether the patient has consulted his/her doctor about the symptoms and, if so, what they were told. A history of travel abroad and gastroenteritis sometimes appears to trigger an irritable bowel. Referral is necessary to exclude an unresolved infection. Any history of previous bowel surgery would suggest a need for referral.

Aggravating factors

Stress appears to play an important role and can precipitate and exacerbate symptoms.

Caffeine often worsens symptoms and its stimulant effect on the bowel and irritant effect on the stomach are well-known in any case.

The sweeteners sorbitol and fructose have also been reported to aggravate IBS. Other foods which have been implicated are milk and dairy products, chocolate, onions, garlic, chives and leeks.

Medication

The patient may already have tried prescribed or over-the-counter (OTC) medicines to treat the condition. You need to know what has been tried and whether it produced any improvement.

It is also important to know what other medicines the patient is taking. Irritable bowel syndrome is associated with anxiety and depression in many patients but it is not known whether this is cause or effect.

When to refer

Children
Older person with no previous history of IBS
Pregnant women
Blood in stools
Unexplained weight loss
Caution in patients aged over 45 with changed bowel habit
Signs of bowel obstruction
Unresponsive to appropriate treatment

Treatment timescale

Symptoms should start to improve within a week.

Management

Antispasmodics

Antispasmodics are the mainstay of OTC treatment of IBS. *Alverine*

---

citrate, peppermint and *mebeverine* are used. They work by a direct effect on the smooth muscle of the gut, causing relaxation and thus reducing abdominal pain. The patient should see an improvement within a few days of starting treatment and should be asked to return to you in a week so you can monitor progress. It is worth trying a different antispasmodic if the first has not worked. Side effects from antispasmodics are rare.

All antispasmodics are contra-indicated in paralytic ileus, a serious condition which fortunately occurs only rarely (after abdominal operations and in peritonitis, for example). Here the gut is not functioning and is obstructed. The symptoms would be severe pain, no bowel movements and possibly vomiting of partly digested food. Immediate referral is needed.

Alverine citrate

This is given in a dose of 60–120 mg (one or two capsules) up to three times a day. Remind the patient to take the capsules with water and not to chew them. Side effects are rare but nausea, dizziness, pruritus, rash and headache have occasionally been reported. The drug should not be recommended for pregnant or breastfeeding women or for children. *Alverine citrate* is also available in a combination product with sterculia (see *Bulking agents,* below).

Peppermint oil

This has been used for many years as an aid to digestion and has an antispasmodic effect. Capsules containing 0.2 ml of the oil are taken in a dose of one or two capsules three times a day, 15 to 30 minutes before meals. They are enteric coated with the intention that the *peppermint oil* is delivered beyond the stomach and upper small bowel. Patients should be reminded not to chew the capsules as not only will this render the treatment ineffective, it will also cause irritation of the mouth and oesophagus.

This treatment should not be recommended for children. Occasionally *peppermint oil* causes heartburn and so is best avoided in patients who already suffer from this problem. Allergic reactions can occur and are rare; rash, headache and muscle tremor have been reported in such cases.

Mebeverine hydrochloride

This was transferred from prescription only medicine (POM) to pharmacy medicine (P) in late 1996 at a dose of 135 mg three times a day. The dose should be taken 20 minutes before meals. The drug should not be recommended for pregnant or breastfeeding women, for children under 10 years of age or for patients with porphyria. *Mebeverine* is also available in a combination product with ispaghula (see *Bulking agents,* below).

Bulking agents

Traditionally patients with IBS were told to eat a diet high in fibre and raw wheat bran was often recommended as a way of increasing the fibre intake. Bran is no longer recommended in IBS (see *Practical Points, Diet*). Bulking agents such as *ispaghula* containing soluble fibre can help some patients. It may take some weeks of experimentation to find the dose which suits the individual patient. Remind the patient that they need to increase their fluid intake to take account of the additional fibre. Bulking agents are also available in combination with antispasmodics.

Antidiarrhoeals

Patients who complain of diarrhoea may be describing a frequent urge to pass stools, but the stools may be loose and formed rather than watery. Use of OTC antidiarrhoeals such as *loperamide* is appropriate only on an occasional, short-term basis.

Practical points

Diet

Patients with IBS should follow the recommendations for a healthy diet (low fat, low sugar, high fibre). Bran used to be widely recommended but more recent research indicates that consumption of bran (which contains insoluble fibre) is not helpful and can make symptoms worse. Dietary sources of soluble fibre can be recommended including oats and pulses.

Some patients find that excluding foods which they know exacerbate their symptoms is helpful (see *Aggravating factors,* above). The sweeteners sorbitol and fructose can make symptoms worse and they are found in many foods: checking labels at the supermarket is needed by patients. Cutting out caffeine, milk and dairy products and chocolate may be worth trying. Although some patients benefit from withdrawal of milk and dairy products there is no evidence of lactase deficiency in IBS. Remind patients that caffeine is included in many soft drinks and so they should check labels.

Complementary therapies

Some patients find relaxation techniques helpful. Videos and audio-cassette tapes are available to teach these.

Studies have shown that hypnotherapy is of benefit in IBS. If the patient wants to try this they should consult a registered hypnotherapist. Others may benefit from traditional acupuncture, reflexology aroma-therapy or homeopathy.

Irritable bowel syndrome in practice

Case 1

Joanna Mathers is a 29-year-old woman who asks to speak to the pharmacist. She has seen an advertisement for an antispasmodic for IBS and wonders whether she should try it. On questioning she tells you that she has been getting stomach pains and bowel symptoms for several months, two or three times a month. She thinks her symptoms seem to be associated with business lunches and dinners at important meetings and include abdominal pain, a feeling of abdominal fullness, diarrhoea, nausea and sometimes vomiting. In answer to your specific question about morning symptoms, Joanna says that sometimes she feels the need to go to the toilet first thing in the morning and may have to go several times. Sometimes she has been late for work because she felt she couldn't leave the house because of the diarrhoea. Joanna tells you that she works as a marketing executive and that her job is pressurized and stressful when there are big deadlines or client meetings. Joanna drinks six or seven cups of coffee a day and says her diet is, 'whatever I can get at work and something from the freezer when I get home'. She is not taking any other medicines and has not been to see the doctor about her problem—she didn't want to bother him.

The pharmacist's view

The picture that has emerged indicates IBS. She has the key symptoms and there is a link to stress at work. It would be worth trying an antispasmodic (*alverine*, *peppermint oil* or *mebeverine*) for a week and asking Joanna to come back at the end of that time. She also needs a careful explanation of aggravating factors for IBS and might want to try a gradual reduction in her intake of coffee over the next few days. If there is no improvement a different antispasmodic could be tried for a further week, with referral then if needed.

The doctor's view

Joanna gives a clear history of IBS. Her symptoms are likely to settle with the pharmacist's advice and treatment. There is up to a 60% placebo response rate in IBS sufferers so it would be surprising if she did not improve when next reviewed. If there was no improvement then a referral would be sensible. A referral would give her doctor an opportunity to deal with her concerns about what was wrong and give her an appropriate explanation of IBS. She could also be given some time to consider how she might tackle her work pressures.

Case 2

Jane Dawson asks to see the pharmacist. She is in her early twenties and says she has been getting some upper abdominal pain after food. She wants to try a stomach medicine. On further questioning she says that she has had an irritable bowel before but this is different, although she does admit that her bowels have been troublesome recently and she has noticed some urinary frequency. Jane says that she has been constipated and felt bloated. She says that she went to her doctor last year and was told she had IBS. The doctor said it was all due to stress which had upset her. Over the last year she has started a new job and moved into new accommodation. She eats a healthy diet and exercises regularly.

The pharmacist's view

The history here is not straightforward and although Jane's symptoms are indicative of IBS, which she says has had before, the symptoms are different on this occasion. The best course of action is to refer her to the doctor for further investigation.

The doctor's view

Jane probably has IBS but there is insufficient information so far to make that diagnosis. It is not uncommon to have upper abdominal pain with IBS, but other possibilities need to be considered. It sounds as though Jane thinks it is coming from her stomach. She may fear that she has an ulcer. She also mentions urinary frequency which may well be associated with IBS but could be an urinary infection. A referral to her doctor is sensible to make a complete assessment of her symptoms. It is likely that the assessment would just involve listening to her description of her problem, gathering more information and a brief examination of her abdomen. A urine sample would show whether or not she had an urinary infection. If there was still doubt about the diagnosis a referral to a gastroenterologist at the local hospital could be made. Between 20 and 50% of referrals to gastroenterologists turn out to be due to IBS. The main purpose of referral is for a diagnosis as there is no therapeutic advantage.

If the doctor thinks Jane has IBS then an explanation of the syndrome would be helpful in addition to dealing with her concerns about a stomach ulcer. Whether or not psychological factors cause IBS there is no doubt that the stresses of life can aggravate symptoms. It therefore makes sense to help sufferers make this connection so they can consider different ways of dealing with stress.

Often the above approach is effective treatment in itself. However, if she did want some medication a bulk bowel regulator to help her constipation plus some antispasmodic tablets would be of value.

Haemorrhoids

Haemorrhoids (commonly known as 'piles') can produce symptoms of itching, burning, pain, swelling and discomfort in the perianal area and anal canal and rectal bleeding. Haemorrhoids are swollen veins, rather like varicose veins, which protrude into the anal canal (internal piles). They may swell so much that they hang down outside the anus (external piles). Haemorrhoids are often caused or exacerbated by inadequate dietary fibre or fluid intake. The pharmacist must, by careful questioning, differentiate between this minor condition and others which may be potentially more serious.

What you need to know
Duration and previous history
Symptoms
Itching, burning
Soreness
Swelling
Pain
Blood in stools
Constipation
Bowel habit
Pregnancy
Other symptoms
Abdominal pain/vomiting
Weight loss
Medication

Significance of questions and answers

Duration and previous history

As an arbitrary guide, the pharmacist might consider treating haemorrhoids of up to 3 weeks' duration. It would be useful to establish whether the patient has a previous history of haemorrhoids and if the doctor has been seen about the problem. A recent examination by the doctor which has excluded serious symptoms would indicate that treatment of symptoms by the pharmacist would be appropriate.

Symptoms

The term haemorrhoids includes 'internal' and 'external' piles, which can be further classified as: those which are confined to the anal canal and cannot be seen; those which prolapse through the anal sphincter on defaecation, then reduce by themselves or are pushed back through the sphincter after defaecation by the patient; and those haemorrhoids which remain persistently prolapsed and outside the anal canal. These three types are sometimes referred to as first, second and third degree respectively. Predisposing factors for haemorrhoids include diet, sedentary occupation and pregnancy and there is thought to be a genetic element.

Pain

Pain is not always present; if it is, it may take the form of a dull ache and may be worse when the patient is having a bowel movement. A severe, sharp pain on defaecation may indicate the presence of an anal fissure, which can have an associated sentinel pile (a small skin tag at the posterior margin of the anus) and requires referral. A fissure is a minute tear in the skin of the anal canal. It is usually caused by constipation and can often be managed conservatively by correcting this and using a local anaesthetic-containing cream or gel. In severe cases a minor operation is sometimes necessary.

Irritation

The most trouble symptom for many patients is itching and irritation of the perianal area rather than pain. Persistent or recurrent irritation which does not improve is sometimes associated with rectal cancer and should be referred.

Bleeding

Blood may be deposited onto the stool from internal haemorrhoids as the stool passes through the anal canal. This fresh blood will appear bright red. It is typically describe as being splashed around the toilet pan and may be seen on the surface of the stool or on the toilet paper. If blood is mixed with the stool, it must have come from higher up the gastrointestinal (GI) tract, and will be dark in colour (altered). If rectal bleeding is present, the pharmacist would be well advised to suggest that the patient sees the doctor so that an examination can be performed to exclude more serious pathology such as tumour or polyps. Colorectal cancer can cause rectal bleeding. The disease is unusual in patients aged under 50 and the pharmacist should be alert for the middle-aged patient with rectal bleeding. This is particularly so if there has been a significant and sustained alteration in bowel habit.

Constipation

Constipation is a common causatory or exacerbatory factor in haemorrhoids. Insufficient dietary fibre and inadequate fluid intake may be involved, although the pharmacist should also consider the possibility of drug-induced constipation.

Straining at stool will occur if the patient is constipated; this increases the pressure in the haemorrhoidal blood vessels in the anal canal and haemorrhoids may result. If piles are painful, the patient may try to avoid defaecation and ignoring the call to open the bowels will make the constipation worse.

Bowel habit

A persisting change in bowel habit is an indication for referral, as it may be caused by a bowel cancer. Seepage of faecal material through the anal sphincter (one form of faecal incontinence) can produce irritation and itching of the perianal area and may be caused by the presence of a tumour.

Pregnancy

Pregnant women have a higher incidence of haemorrhoids than non-pregnant women. This is thought to be due to pressure on the haemorrhoidal vessels due to the gravid uterus. Constipation in pregnancy is also a common problem because raised progesterone levels mean that the gut muscles tend to be more relaxed. Such constipation can exacerbate symptoms of haemorrhoids. Appropriate dietary advice can be offered by the pharmacist.

Other symptoms

Symptoms of haemorrhoids remain 'local' to the anus. They do not cause abdominal pain, distension or vomiting. Any of these more 'widespread' symptoms suggest other problems and require referral.

Tenesmus (the desire to defaecate when there is no stool present in the rectum) sometimes occurs when there is a tumour in the rectum. The patient may describe a feeling of often wanting to pass a motion but no faeces being present.

Medication

Patients may already have tried one or more proprietary preparations to treat their symptoms. Some of these products are advertised widely, since the problem of haemorrhoids is perceived as potentially embarrassing and such advertisements may sometimes discourage patients from describing their symptoms. It is therefore important for the pharmacist to identify the exact nature of the symptoms being experienced and details of any products used already. If the patient is constipated, the use of any laxatives should be established.

Present medication
Haemorrhoids may be exacerbated by drug-induced constipation and the patient should be carefully questioned about current medication, including prescription and over-the-counter (OTC) medicines. A list of drugs which may cause constipation can be found on p. 94. Rectal bleeding in a patient taking *warfarin* or another anticoagulant is an indication for referral.

p. 94

When to refer

Duration of longer than 3 weeks
Presence of blood in the stools
Change in bowel habit (persisting alteration from normal bowel habit)
Suspected drug-induced constipation
Associated abdominal pain/vomiting

Treatment timescale

If symptoms have not improved after a week, patients should see their doctor.

Management

Symptomatic treatment of haemorrhoids can provide relief from discomfort but if present, the underlying cause of constipation must also be addressed. The pharmacist is in a good position to offer dietary advice, in addition to treatment, to prevent recurrent of symptoms in the future.

Local anaesthetics (e.g. *benzocaine, lignocaine*)
These can help to reduce the pain and itching associated with haemorrhoids. There is a possibility that local anaesthetics may cause sensitization and their use is best limited to a maximum of 2 weeks.

Skin protectors
Many antihaemorrhoidal products are bland, soothing preparations containing skin protectors (e.g. *zinc oxide* and *kaolin*). These products have emollient and protective properties. Protection of the perianal skin is important, because the presence of faecal matter can cause symptoms

such as irritation and itching. Protecting agents form a barrier on the skin surface, helping to prevent irritation and loss of moisture from the skin.

Topical steroids

Ointment and suppositories containing hydrocortisone with skin protectors, previously prescription only medicines (POM), are now available OTC. The steroid reduces inflammation and swelling to give relief from itching and pain. The treatment should be used each morning and at night and after a bowel movement. The use of such products is restricted to those aged over 18. Treatment should not be used continuously for longer than seven days.

Astringents

Astringents such as *zinc oxide, hamamelis* (witch hazel) and *bismuth salts* are included in products on the theoretical basis that they will cause precipitation of proteins when applied to mucous membranes or skin which is broken or damaged. A protective layer is then thought to be formed, helping to relieve irritation and inflammation. Some astringents also have a protective and mild antiseptic action, (e.g. *bismuth*).

Antiseptics

These are among the ingredients of many antihaemorrhoidal products, including the medicated toilet tissues. They do not have a specific action in the treatment of haemorrhoids. *Resorcinol* has antiseptic, antipruritic and exfoliative properties. The exfoliative action is thought to be useful by removing the top layer of skin cells and aiding penetration of medicaments into the skin. *Resorcinol* can be absorbed systemically via broken skin if there is prolonged use and its antithyroid action can lead to the development of myxoedema (hypothyroidism).

Counter-irritants

Counter-irritants such as *menthol* are sometimes included in antihaemorrhoidal products on the basis that their stimulation of nerve endings gives a sensation of cooling and tingling which distracts from the sensation of pain. *Menthol* and *phenol* also have antipruritic actions.

Shark liver oil/live yeast

These agents are said to promote healing and tissue repair, but there is no scientific evidence to support such claims.

Laxatives

The short-term use of a laxative to relieve constipation might be considered. One or 2 days' supply of a stimulant laxative (e.g. *senna*) should help to deal with the immediate problem while dietary fibre and fluids are being increased. For patients who cannot or choose not to adapt their diet, bulk laxatives may be used long term.

Practical points

Self-diagnosis

Patients may say that they have piles, or think they have piles, but careful questioning by the pharmacist is needed to check whether this self-diagnosis is correct. If there is any doubt, referral is the best course of action.

Hygiene

The itching of haemorrhoids can often be improved by good anal hygiene, since the presence of small amounts of faecal matter can cause itching to occur. The perianal area should be washed with warm water as frequently as is practicable, ideally after each bowel movement. Soap will tend to dry the skin and could make itching worse, but a mild soap could be tried if the patient wishes to do so. Moist toilet tissues are available and these can be very useful where washing is not practical, for example, at work during the daytime, and some patients prefer them. These tissues are better used with a patting rather than a rubbing motion, which might aggravate symptoms. Many people with haemorrhoids find that a warm bath soothes their discomfort.

An increased intake of dietary fibre will increase bowel output, so that patients can be well advised to take care in wiping the perianal area and to use soft toilet paper to avoid soreness after wiping.

How to use over-the-counter products

Ointments and creams can be used for internal and external haemorrhoids and should be applied in the morning at night and after each bowel movement. An applicator is included in packs of ointment and creams and patients should be advised to take care in its use, to avoid any further damage to the perianal skin

Suppositories can be recommended for internal haemorrhoids. After removing the foil or plastic packaging (patients have been known to try and insert them with the packaging left on), a suppository should be inserted morning, night and after bowel movements. Insertion is easier if the patient is crouching or lying down.

Haemorrhoids in practice

Case 1

Tom Harris, a customer whom you know quite well, asks if you can recommend something for his 'usual problem'. You ask him to tell you more about it: Mr Harris suffers from piles occasionally; you have dispensed prescriptions for Anusol HC and similar products in the past; and have previously advised him about dietary fibre and fluid intake. He has been away on holiday for 2 weeks and says he hasn't been eating the same foods he does when at home. His symptoms are itching and irritation of the perianal area but no pain and he has a small swelling, which hangs down from the anus after he has passed a motion but which he is able to push back again. He is a little constipated, but is not taking any medicines.

The pharmacist's view

Mr Harris has a previous history of haemorrhoids, which have been diagnosed and treated by his doctor. It is likely that his holiday and temporary change in diet have caused a recurrence of the problem, so that he now has a second degree pile, and it would be reasonable to suggest symptomatic treatment for a few days. You could recommend the use of an ointment preparation containing *hydrocortisone* and skin protectors for up to a week, and remind Mr Harris that the area should be kept clean and dry. You might consider recommending a laxative to ease the constipation until Mr Harris's diet gets back to normal (you advise that he returns to his usual high-fibre diet); a small supply of a stimulant laxative (perhaps a stimulant/stool softener such as docusate sodium) would be reasonable. He should see his doctor after a week if the problem has not cleared up.

The doctor's view

The treatment suggested by the pharmacist should settle Mr Harris's symptoms within a week. The treatment is of course symptomatic and not curative. If he continues to suffer from frequent relapse, referral should be considered. His doctor could advise whether or not to refer him for injection or removal of the piles.

Case 2

Mr Briggs is a local shopkeeper in his late fifties who wants you to recommend something for his piles. He tells you that he has had them for quite a while—a couple of months. He has tried several different ointments and suppositories, all to no avail. The main problem now is bleeding, which has became worse. In fact he tells you, somewhat embarrassed, that he has been buying sanitary towels because this is the only way he can prevent his clothes from becoming stained. He is not constipated and has no pain.

The pharmacist's view

Mr Briggs should be referred to his doctor at once. His symptoms have a history of 2 months and there must be quite profuse rectal bleeding, which may well be due to a more serious disease. He has already tried some OTC treatments, with no success. His age and the description of his symptoms mean that further investigation is needed.

The doctor's view

Mr Briggs should be advised to see his doctor. This is not a typical presentation of piles. He will need a more detailed assessment by his doctor who will need to look for a cancer of the colon or rectum. Piles can bleed at times other than when defaecating but this is uncommon. The doctor would gather more information by questioning and from an examination. The examination would usually include a digital rectal assessment to determine whether or not a rectal tumour is present. It is quite likely that this man would require out-patient hospital referral for further investigations which would involve sigmoidoscopy and barium enema.

Case 3

Caroline Andrews is a young woman in her mid twenties, who works as a graphic designer in a local art studio. She asks your advice about an embarrassing problem: she is finding it very painful to pass motions. On questioning, she tells you she has had the problem for a few days and has been constipated for about 2 weeks. She eats a diet which sounds relatively low in fibre and has been eating less than usual because she has been very busy at work. Caroline says she seldom takes any exercise. She takes the contraceptive pill but is not taking any medicines and has no other symptoms such as rectal bleeding.

The pharmacist's view

Caroline would probably be best advised to see her doctor, since the symptoms and pain which she has described might be due to an anal fissure, though they may be caused by a haemorrhoid.

The doctor's view

A fissure would be the most likely cause of Caroline's problem. An examination by her doctor should quickly confirm this. Correction of the constipation and future preventative dietary advice could well solve the problem. The discomfort could be helped by a local anaesthetic-containing cream or gel. If this is applied prior to a bowel action, the discomfort would be less. Occasionally, when the symptoms are severe, referral to a surgeon is best as a simple procedure to release the excess spasm in the anal sphincter under general anaesthesia will produce rapid relief of pain.

Skin Conditions

Eczema/dermatitis

Eczema is a term used synomously with dermatitis. The latter is more correctly used when an external precipitating factor is present (contact dermatitis). The rashes produced have similar features but the distribution on the body varies and can be diagnostic.

The rash of eczema typically presents as dry flaky skin which may be inflamed and have small red spots. The skin may be cracked and weepy and sometimes becomes thickened. The rash is irritant and can be extremely itchy.

> **What you need to know**
>
> Age
> Distribution of rash
> Occupation/contact
> Previous history
> History of hay fever/asthma
> Aggravating factors
> Medication

Significance of questions and answers

Age/distribution

The distribution of the rash tends to vary with age. In infants, it is usually present around the nappy area, neck and back of scalp, face, limb creases and backs of the wrists.

In children, the rash is most marked behind the knees, on the inside of the elbow joint, on the hands, around the wrists, ankles, neck and eyes.

In adults, the neck, the backs of the hands, the groin, around the anus, the ankles and feet are the most common sites. The rash of intertrigo is caused by a fungal infection and is found in skin folds or occluded areas such as under the breasts in women and in the groin or armpits.

Occupation/contact

Contact dermatitis may be caused by substances which irritate the skin or which spark off an allergic reaction. Substances which can irritate the skin include: alkaline cleansing agents; degreasing agents; solvents and oils; and oxidizing and reducing agents (e.g. as used by hairdressers when perming hair). Such substances either cause direct and rapid damage to the skin or, in the case of weaker irritants, exert their irritant effect after continued exposure. Classic examples of irritant dermatitis include 'housewives' eczema', due to continued exposure to detergents and wetting, and napkin dermatitis.

In other cases the contact dermatitis is caused by an allergic response to substances which include chromates (present in cement and rust-preventive paint), nickel (e.g. in costume jewellery and as plating on scissors), rubber and resins (two-part glues and the resin colophony in adhesive plasters), dyes and certain plants (e.g. primula). Eye make-up and jewellery can also cause allergic contact dermatitis.

Clues as to whether or not a contact problem is present can be gleaned from knowledge of: site of rash; details of job and hobbies; onset of rash and agents handled; and improvement of rash when away from work or on holiday.

Previous history

Patients may ask the pharmacist to recommend treatment for eczema which has been diagnosed by the doctor. In cases of mild eczema, it would be reasonable for the pharmacist to recommend the use of emollients and to advise on skin care. However, where exacerbations of eczema have occured, the patient is best referred to the doctor. *Topical hydrocortisone* preparations can be recommended for the treatment of mild to moderate eczema.

Occasionally, pharmacists receive requests for *topical hydrocortisone* products from patients on the recommendation of their doctors. It can be difficult to explain why such a sale cannot be made if the product is for use on the face or anogenital area or for severe eczema. Pharmacists can minimize such problems by ensuring that local family doctors (especially trainees) are aware of the restrictions which apply to the sale of *hydrocortisone* over the counter (OTC).

History of hay fever/asthma

Many eczema sufferers have associated hay fever and/or asthma. There is often a family history of eczema, hay fever or asthma. Eczema occurring in such situations is called atopic eczema. The pharmacist can enquire during questioning about family history of these conditions.

Aggravating factors

Atopic eczema may be worsened during the hay fever season and by house dust or animal danders. Factors which dry the skin such as soaps or detergents and cold wind can aggravate. Certain clothing such as woollen material can irritate. In a small minority of sufferers (less than 5%) cow's milk, eggs and food colouring (tartrazine) have been implicated. Emotional factors, stress and worry can sometimes exacerbate eczema. Antiseptic solutions applied directly to the skin or added to the bath water can irritate the skin.

Medication

Contact dermatitis may be caused or made worse by sensitization to topical medicaments. The pharmacist should ask which treatments have already been used. Topically applied local anaesthetics, antihistamines, antibiotics and antiseptics can all provoke allergic dermatitis. Lanolin has been a common cause of allergic reactions and is present in many OTC treatments, cosmetic moisturizers and hand creams. More highly purified lanolin is now available, but sensitization problems have not been entirely eradicated. Some preservatives may cause sensitization. Information about different preparations and their formulations can be obtained from the local drug information pharmacist or from the manufacturer of the product. The *British National Formulary* is also a good source of information on this subject, with additives listed for each topical product.

If the patient has used a preparation which the pharmacist considers appropriate for the condition but there has been no improvement or the condition has worsened, the patient should see the doctor.

When to refer
Evidence of infection (weeping)
Severe condition; badly fissured/cracked skin, bleeding
Failed medication
No identifiable cause (unless previously diagnosed as eczema)
Duration of longer than 2 weeks

Treatment timescale

Irritant and allergic dermatitis should respond to skin care and treatment with OTC products. If no improvement has been noted after a week, referral to the doctor is advisable.

Management

Skin rashes tend quite understandably to cause much anxiety. There is also a social stigma associated with skin disease. Many patients will therefore have been seen by their doctor. Pharmacists are most likely to be involved where the diagnosis has already been made, or when the condition first presents but is very mild.

However, as much of the management involves advice and the use of emollients, the pharmacist is in a good position to help. Where the pharmacist is able to identify a cause of irritant or allergic dermatitis, *topical hydrocortisone* may be recommended.

Emollients

These are the key to managing eczema and are medically inert creams and ointments which can be used to: soothe the skin; reduce irritation; prevent the skin from drying; act as a protective layer; and be used as a soap substitute. They may be applied directly to the skin or added to the bath water. Proprietary general-purpose emollient creams and ointments should be used as often as needed. Adding *Emulsifying ointment* or a proprietary bath oil to the bath is helpful. *Emulsifying ointment* should first be mixed with water (1 or 2 tablespoonfuls of ointment in a bowl of hot water) before being added to the bath to ensure distribution in the bathwater. Some patients with eczema believe, incorrectly, that bathing will make their eczema worse. This is not the case providing appropriate emollient products are used and standard soaps and perfumed bath products are avoided.

There are many different types of emollient preparation which vary in their degree of greasiness. The greasy preparations such as *white soft paraffin* are often the most effective, especially with very dry skin, but have the disadvantage of being messy and unpleasant to use. Patient preference is very important and plays a major part in compliance with emollient treatments.

Emollient preparations should be used as often as is needed to keep the skin hydrated and moist. Several and frequent applications each day may be required to achieve this.

Advice

This could include the identification of possible aggravating or precipitating factors. If the history is suggestive of an occupationally associated contact dermatitis, then referral is advisable. The doctor may feel in turn that referral to a dermatologist is appropriate. It is sometimes necessary for a specialist to perform patch testing to identify the cause of contact dermatitis.

Further advice could be given regarding the use of ordinary soaps, which tend to dry the skin and their alternatives (soap substitutes).

If steroid creams have been prescribed and emollients are to be used, the pharmacist is in a good position to check that the patient understands the way in which they should be used.

Topical hydrocortisone

Hydrocortisone cream and *ointment* can be sold OTC for a limited range of indications: irritant and allergic dermatitis; insect bites; and mild to moderate eczema. Over-the-counter *hydrocortisone* is contra-indicated where the skin is infected (e.g. athlete's foot or cold sores), in acne and on the face and anogenital areas. Only adults and children over 10 years of age can be treated and any course must not be longer than 1 week. Only proprietary OTC brands of *topical hydrocortisone* can be used; dispensing packs may not be sold.

Antipruritics

Antipruritic preparations are sometimes useful. *Aqueous calamine cream* is extremely useful for this purpose and its effectiveness is increased by adding *1% menthol* to give additional antipruritic and cooling actions.

Crotamiton is an excellent agent for reducing the discomfort of itchy skin and is available in cream and lotion forms. A combination product containing *crotamiton with hydrocortisone* has been deregulated from prescription only control and can be sold OTC. Indications for use are the same as for *topical hydrocortisone*—contact dermatitis (irritant or allergic), insect bites or stings and mild to moderate eczema. The same restrictions on use apply (see *Topical hydrocortisone* above).

Eczema and dermatitis in practice

Case 1

Lesley Tibbs is a young mother who had her first baby a few weeks ago. She asks your advice about her hands which are dry and sore. The skin is flaky but not broken and there is no sign of secondary infection such as weeping or pus. Only the skin of the hands is affected. Mrs Tibbs has occasionally had the problem before but not so severely. On further questioning, you discover that she is soaking terry nappies in a proprietary solution before putting them in a washing machine. She does not wear gloves. She has not changed her detergent or washing powder and she has no history of hay fever or asthma.

The pharmacist's view

Mrs Tibbs has an irritant contact dermatitis caused by the chemicals (soaking solution for nappies and detergent) which her hands are coming into contact with. It is exacerbated by repeated wetting of the skin. *Hydrocortisone ointment* could be recommended for 1 week and additional emollient preparation may also be useful. The *hydrocortisone ointment* should be applied sparingly twice daily and the emollient as often as needed. If the skin is very itchy, *crotamiton with hydrocortisone* could be recommended. You could ask her to call back and see you in 2 week's time to report progress. It is important that this lady understands the cause of the problem and that the skin should be protected against detergents and wetting by wearing rubber gloves.

The doctor's view

The pharmacist's assessment and recommendations are correct. It is not uncommon for contact dermatitis to persist for longer than a week despite the above measures. If this is so, referral to the doctor may be advisable. Skin disorders often cause much anxiety. This may be particularly relevant for Mrs Tibbs who will already be stressed by recently having her first baby. The stress may even be a contributory factor in her skin problem. Any anxiety can be helped by finding out what concerns Mrs Tibbs and how much she understands about her problem, for example; 'Is it infectious? Can I give it to my baby? Will it spread?'. Once her concerns have been listened to, any factual errors can be corrected and further information given. At this stage the doctor could then ask her about her views on management, which might include any concerns she may have about the use of topical steroids. Many people are aware that 'steroids' can have serious side effects. Thus it can be helpful to explain when steroids can cause problems and their nature. This should then lead to a mutually agreed plan of treatment which, if Mrs Tibbs has been given good information and had her concerns dealt with, should lead to good compliance. If Mrs Tibbs did not understand her treatment or if, for example, she was frightened that steroid cream might be harmful to her or even to her baby, then she would be less likely to use the treatment properly.

Case 2

Ray Timpson is a local man in his mid thirties and a regular customer. Today he wants to buy some *hydrocortisone cream* for his eczema which has flared up. He has had eczema for many years and usually obtains his *hydrocortisone cream* on a repeat prescription from his doctor. As a child Mr Timpson was asthmatic and both asthma and hay fever are present in some members of his family. He has just seen an advert for a proprietary OTC *hydrocortisone cream* and says he would prefer to buy his supplies from you in the future to save both himself and the doctor some time The eczema affects his ankles, shins and hands; the skin on his hands is cracked and weeping.

The pharmacist's view

Mr Timpson needs to see his doctor because the eczema on his hands is infected. Topical steroids, including *hydrocortisone*, should not be used on infected skin.

The doctor's view

One reason why pharmacists were not initially allowed to sell OTC *hydrocortisone* in eczema is because it may have to be used by some people for many months or years at a time. It is sensible practice for the doctor to review patients on long-term repeat prescriptions from time to time. Practically, however, *hydrocortisone cream* is safe providing the contra-indications are observed. A review by the doctor would provide an opportunity to reassess the appropriateness of treatment. In this case it would be necessary to check out Mr Timpson's understanding of his problem. It would be helpful to clarify what else helps his skin and whether he uses an emollient. Once further information has been obtained a future plan can be decided upon. The infection would need to be treated. It might be appropriate in some patients to use a potent topical steroid for a short period to control symptoms, rather than persisting with a weaker one in the long term.

Acne

The incidence of acne in teenagers is extremely high and it has been estimated that over half of all adolescents will experience some degree of acne. Most acne sufferers resort, at least initially, to self-treatment. Mild acne often responds well to correctly used over-the-counter (OTC) treatments. Pharmacists should remember that self-conscious teenagers regard acne as a major problem and that a sympathetic response to requests for help, together with an invitation to return and report progress, can be as important as the treatment selected.

What you need to know
Age
Severity
Mild, moderate, severe
Affected areas
Duration
Medication

Significance of questions and answers

Age

Acne commonly occurs during the teenage years and its onset is most common at puberty, although it may start to appear a year or so before puberty. Acne can persist for anything from a few months to several years; with onset at puberty, acne may continue until the late teens or even early twenties. The hormonal changes which occur during puberty, especially the production of androgens, are thought to be involved in the causation of acne. Increased keratin and sebum production during adolescence are thought to be important contributory factors; the increased amount of keratin leads to blockages of the follicles and the formation of comedones (a comedone is a mass of keratin and sebum).

Very young

Acne is extremely rare in young children and babies and any such cases should be referred to the doctor for further investigation since an androgen-secreting (hormone-producing) tumour may be responsible.

Older

For patients in whom acne begins later than the teenage years, other causes should be considered, including drug therapy (discussed below) and occupational factors. Oils and greases used at work can precipitate acne and it would be worth asking whether the patient comes into contact with such agents. Acne worsens just before or during menstruation in some women; this is thought to be due to changes in progesterone levels.

Severity

Over-the-counter treatment may be recommended for mild acne. Comedones may be 'open' or 'closed', the sebum in closed comedones cannot reach the surface of the skin. The plug of keratin which is at the entrance to the follicle in a comedone is initially white (a whitehead), later becoming darker coloured because of the accumulation of melanin (a blackhead). However, sebum is still produced, so that swelling occurs and the comedone eventually ruptures, discharging its contents under the skin's surface. The released sebum causes an inflammatory response; if the response is not severe, small red papules appear. In more severe acne, angry-looking red pustules are seen and referral to the doctor for alternative forms of treatment such as topical or systemic antibiotics is needed.

Affected areas

In acne these may include the face, neck, centre of the chest, upper back and shoulders; all areas with large numbers of sebaceous glands. Rosacea is a skin condition which is sometimes confused with acne. Occurring in young and middle-aged adults, rosacea has characteristic features of reddening, papules and pustules. Only the face is affected.

Duration

The information gained here should be considered in conjunction with facts about medication (prescribed or OTC) tried already and about other medicines being taken. Acne of long duration where several OTC preparations had been correctly used without success would indicate referral to the doctor.

Medication

The pharmacist should establish the identity of any treatment tried already and its method of use. Inappropriate use of medication, for example infrequent application, could affect the chances of success.

Information about current therapy is important, since acne can sometimes be drug induced. *Lithium, phenytoin* and progestogens (e.g.

in the oral contraceptive pill) may be culprits. If acne is suspected as a result of drug therapy, patients should be advised to discuss this with their doctor.

When to refer

Acne in the very young
Severe acne
Failed medication
Suspected drug-induced acne

Treatment timescale

A patient with mild acne which has not responded to treatment within 8 weeks should be referred to the doctor.

Management

Dozens of products are marketed for the treatment of acne. The pharmacist can make a logical selection based on knowledge of likely efficacy. The general aims of therapy are to remove follicular plugs so that sebum is able to flow freely and to reduce the number of bacteria on the skin. Treatment should therefore reduce comedone formation. The most useful formulations are lotions, creams and gels. Gels with an alcoholic base dry quickly but can be irritant. Those with an aqueous base dry more slowly but are less likely to irritate the skin.

Benzoyl peroxide

Benzoyl peroxide is the first-line OTC treatment for acne. It has a keratolytic action, which increases the turnover of skin cells, helping the skin to peel and also antibacterial properties, which should help to reduce the skin flora. Regular application can result in improvement of mild acne. At first, *benzoyl peroxide* is very likely to produce reddening and soreness of the skin and patients should be warned of this (see *Practical points* below). Treatment should start with a 2.5 or 5% product, moving gradually to the 10% strength.

Sensitization

Occasionally, sensitization to *benzoyl peroxide* may occur. The skin becomes reddened, inflamed and sore, and treatment should be discontinued.

Bleaching

Warning should be given that *benzoyl peroxide* can bleach clothing and bedding. If it is applied at night, white sheets and pillowcases are best used and patients can be advised to wear an old T-shirt or shirt to minimize damage to good clothes. Contact between *benzoyl peroxide* and the eyes, mouth and other mucous membranes should be avoided.

Other keratolytics

These include *potassium hydroxyquinoline sulphate, sulphur, resorcinol* and *salicylic acid. Potassium hydroxyquinoline sulphate* also has antibacterial activity. *Sulphur* has some antiseptic activity in addition to its keratolytic effect. There seems to be evidence that *sulphur* can itself be comedogenic, that is, it can lead to comedone formation, so it would not be considered a first-line treatment. Prolonged application of *resorcinol* can affect thyroid function, so continued use of products containing *resorcinol* is not advisable, though the relative risk in acne is probably small unless large areas of skin are involved. The use of *resorcinol* in black-skinned patients is not advisable because it may least to skin discoloration. *Salicylic acid* has some antibacterial and antifungal actions.

Antibacterials

Skin washes and soaps are available containing antiseptic agents such as *chlorhexidine*. Such products can be useful in acne by degreasing the skin and reducing the skin flora.

One combination product is available containing *benzoyl peroxide* together with *miconazole*, an antifungal agent with antibacterial activity. Such a combination should fulfil both aims of acne treatments—that is, to unblock follicular plugs and reduce the number of bacteria on the skin.

Practical points

Diet

There is absolutely no evidence to link diet with acne, despite a common belief that chocolate and fatty foods cause acne or make it worse.

Sunlight

Ultraviolet light can be helpful in acne and advice can be given to spend more time in the sun. The beneficial effects of sunlight are thought to be due to its peeling effect, which helps unblock follicles, and the drying or degreasing effect of the sun on the skin may also be valuable. The use of artificial forms of ultraviolet light such as sunbeds is not to be encouraged, since evidence suggests that the risk of melanoma is increased.

Keratolytics

All keratolytics make the skin peel and can therefore can be useful in treating acne. They should be applied to the whole of the affected area, not just to individual comedones, and are best applied to skin following washing. During the first few days of use the skin is likely to become reddened and may feel slightly sore. Warning should be given that such an irritant effect is likely to occur, otherwise treatment may be abandoned inappropriately.

One approach to minimize reddening and skin soreness is to begin with the lowest strength preparation and to apply the cream, lotion or gel sparingly and infrequently during the first week of treatment. Once-daily application, or application on alternate days, could be tried for a week and then frequency of use increased. After 2 or 3 weeks a higher strength preparation may be introduced. If irritant effects continue after a week, or are severe, use of the product should be discontinued.

Antibiotics

The pharmacist is in a good position to ensure that acne treatments are used correctly. Oral antibiotic therapy usually consists of tetracyclines and patients should be reminded not to eat or drink dairy products up to an hour before or after taking the antibiotic. The same rule applies to antacid or iron preparations. Evidence suggests that failure of antibiotic therapy in acne in the past may have been due to subclinical levels of antibiotic because of chelation by metal ions in dairy products or antacids.

Continuous treatment

Acne is notoriously slow to respond to treatment and a period of up to 6 months may be required for maximum benefit. It is generally agreed that keratolytics such as *benzoyl peroxide* require a minimum of 6 weeks' treatment for benefit to be shown. Patients should therefore be encouraged to persevere with treatment, whether with OTC or prescription products and told not to feel discouraged if results are not immediate. Research has shown that many teenagers have unrealistic expectations of the time needed for improvement to be seen, perhaps created by the advertising for some treatments. The patient also needs to understand that acne is a chronic condition and that continuous treatment is needed to keep the problem under control.

Skin hygiene

Acne is not caused by poor hygiene, nor by failure to wash the skin sufficiently often. However, regular washing of the skin with soap and warm water, or preferably with an antibacterial soap or skin wash, can be helpful as it degreases the skin and reduces the number of bacteria present.

Facial washes and soap substitutes can sometimes help to motivate patients to wash regularly. Since personal hygiene is a sensitive area, an initial inquiry about the kind of soap or wash currently being used might be a tactful way to introduce the subject. Dermabrasion with facial scrubs can help by removing the outer layer of dead skin but must be done gently. The patient needs to understand that scrubbing harshly will not produce an improved effect.

Topical hydrocortisone and acne

The use of *topical hydrocortisone* is contra-indicated in acne because steroids can potentiate the effects of androgenic hormones on the sebaceous glands, hence making acne worse.

Removal of comedones

Comedone expressors can be bought to remove blackheads; they are applied to the comedone and have a small hole through which the comedone is extracted when pressure is applied. Steam will aid the removal of comedones. However, some dermatologists advise against attempts to remove comedones, because the application of pressure may damage the follicles and also spread sebum and pus to previously unaffected skin areas, leading to infection, inflammation and possible scarring. Certainly the squeezing of comedones and spots with the fingers is to be discouraged for the same reasons.

Make-up

Heavy, greasy make-up can only exacerbate acne. If make-up is to be worn, water-based rather than oily foundations are best and should be removed thoroughly at the end of the day.

Athlete's foot

The incidence of athlete's foot (*Tinea pedis*) is not, as its name might suggest, limited to those of an athletic disposition. The fungus which causes the disease thrives in warm, moist conditions. The spaces between the toes can provide a good growth environment and the infection therefore has a high incidence. The problem is more common in men than in women and responds well to over-the-counter (OTC) treatment.

What you need to know
Duration
Appearance
Severity
Broken skin
Soreness
Secondary infection
Location
Previous history
Medication

Significance of questions and answers

Duration

Considered together with its severity, a long-standing condition may make the pharmacist decide to refer the patient. However, most cases of athlete's foot are minor in nature and can be treated effectively with products available OTC.

Appearance

Athlete's foot usually presents as itchy, flaking skin in the web spaces between the toes. The flakes or scales of skin become white and macerated and begin to peel off. Underneath the scales, the skin is usually reddened and may be itchy and sore. The skin may be dry and scaly or moist and weeping.

Severity

Athlete's foot is usually a mild fungal infection, but occasionally the skin between the toes becomes more macerated and broken and deeper and painful fissures may develop. The skin may then become inflamed and sore. Once the skin is broken, there is the potential for secondary bacterial infection to develop. If there are indications of bacterial involvement—weeping, pus or yellow crusts—referral to the doctor is needed.

Location

Classically the toes are involved, the web space between the fourth and fifth toes being the most affected. More severe infections may spread to the sole of the foot and even to the upper surface in some cases. This type of spread can alter the appearance of the condition and severe cases are probably best referred to the doctor for further investigation. When other areas of the foot are involved, the appearance can be confused with that of allergic dermatitis. However, in eczema or dermatitis, the spaces between the toes are usually spared, in contrast to athlete's foot.

If the toenails appear to be involved, referral to the doctor will be necessary because systemic antifungal treatment may be required to deal with infection of the nail bed. Even with systemic treatment it is not always possible to eradicate such infections.

Previous history

Many people suffer occasionally from athlete's foot. The pharmacist should ask about previous bouts and about the action taken in response. Any diabetic patient who presents with athlete's foot is best referred to the doctor. Diabetics may have impaired circulation or innervation of the feet and are more prone to secondary infections in addition to poorer healing of open wounds.

Medication

One or more topical treatments may have been tried before the patient seeks advice from the pharmacist. The identity of any treatment should be established and the method of use. Treatment failure may occur simply because it was not continued sufficiently long enough. However, if an appropriate antifungal product has been used correctly without remission of symptoms, the patient is best referred to the doctor, especially if the problem is of long duration (several weeks).

When to refer
Severe, affecting other parts of the foot
Signs of bacterial infection
Unresponsive to appropriate treatment
Diabetic patients
Involvement of toenails

Treatment timescale

If athelete's foot has not responded to treatment within 2 weeks patients should see their doctor.

Management

Many preparations are available for the treatment of athelete's foot. Formulations include creams, powders, solutions, sprays and paints. Some older antifungal agents are less effective than those more recently introduced. Pharmacists should instruct patients on how to use the treatment correctly and on other measures which can help to prevent recurrence (see *Practical points* below). Regular application of the recommended product to clean, dry feet is essential and treatment must be continued after symptoms have gone to ensure eradication of the fungus. A minimum of 2–4 weeks treatment is usually needed.

Imidazoles (e.g. *miconazole, clotrimazole*)

The imidazoles are the most effective group of antifungal agents and can be used to treat many topical fungal infections, including athelete's foot, where they are the treatment of choice. Imidazoles have a wide spectrum of action and *miconazole* has been shown to have both antifungal and antibacterial activity. The treatment should be applied two or three times daily. Formulations include creams, powders and sprays. *Miconazole* and *clotrimazole* have occasionally been reported to cause mild irritation of the skin.

Tolnaftate

Tolnaftate is available in powder, cream, aerosol and solution formulations and is effective against athelete's foot. It has antifungal but not antibacterial action. It should be applied twice daily and treatment should be continued for up to 6 weeks. *Tolnaftate* may sting slightly when applied to infected skin. *Tolnaftate* is useful in dry, scaly athelete's foot. Where the skin is soggy and macerated an imidazole is more likely to be effective because of its additional antibacterial action.

Undecenoates (e.g. *zinc undecenoate, undecenoic acid, methyl* and *propyl undecylenate*)

Undecenoic acid is an antifungal agent, sometimes formulated with *zinc salt* to give additional astringent properties. It is effective in mild cases of athelete's foot but less effective than the imidazoles or *tolnaftate*. Treatment should be continued for 4 weeks.

Benzoic acid

Benzoic acid has antifungal properties and is a traditional treatment for athlete's foot. *Whitfield's ointment,* also known as *compound benzoic acid ointment,* contains *benzoic acid* with *salicylic acid.* The rationale for its use is that the keratolytic action of *salicylic acid* exfoliates the upper layers of skin, allowing the antifungal *benzoic acid* to penetrate the infected layers. The effectiveness of *benzoic acid* as an antifungal agent is questionable and the development of the imidazoles has meant that effective antifungals are now available in formulations which are more pleasant to use. *Whitfield's ointment* sometimes stings on application and its formulation is rather greasy. Its use has now been largely superseded by newer products. The same ingredients are now available in a proprietary cream formulation which is more pleasant to use.

Hydrocortisone cream or ointment

Hydrocortisone may be sold OTC for allergic and irritant dermatitis, insect bites or stings and mild to moderate eczema. The pharmacist may not recommend the use of *topical hydrocortisone* in athlete's foot because, although it would reduce inflammation, it would not deal with the fungal infection which might then worsen. Combination products containing *hydrocortisone* together with an antifungal agent are, however, available OTC for use in athlete's foot and intertrigo. Treatment is limited to 7 days.

Practical points

Footwear

Sweating of the feet can produce the kind of hot, moist environment in which the fungus is able to grow. Shoes which are too tight and which are made of synthetic materials make it impossible for moisture to evaporate. If possible, the patient should wear leather shoes, which will allow the skin to 'breathe'. In summer, open-toed sandals can be helpful, and shoes should be left off where possible. The wearing of cotton socks can facilitate the evaporation of moisture, whereas nylon socks will prevent this.

Foot hygiene

The feet should be washed and carefully and thoroughly dried, especially between the toes, before the antifungal preparation is applied.

Transmission of athlete's foot

Athlete's foot is easily transmitted and is thought to be acquired by walking barefoot, for example on changing-room floors in workplaces, schools and sports clubs. The wearing of some form of footwear such as rubber sandals can therefore be useful.

Prevention of reinfection

Care should be taken to ensure that shoes and socks are kept free of the fungus. Socks should be changed and washed regularly. Shoes can be dusted with a fungicidal powder to eradicate the fungus. The use of a fungicidal dusting powder on the feet and in the shoes can be a useful prophylactic measure and can also help to absorb moisture and prevent maceration. Patients should be reminded to treat all shoes, since fungal spores may be present.

Frequency and length of treatment

Products should be applied to clean, dry feet twice daily, in the morning and the evening. Any treatment should be continued for 2 weeks after the symptoms of athlete's foot have disappeared, to ensure that the infection is eradicated. A total treatment time of 2–4 weeks might be expected. If the condition has not improved after 2 weeks, referral to the doctor is advisable.

Ringworm

Ringworm of the body (*Tinea corporis*) is a fungal infection which occurs as a circular lesion that gradually spreads after beginning as a small, red, papule. Often there is only one lesion and the characteristic appearance is of a central, cleared area with a red advancing edge. Topical imidazoles such as *miconazole* are effective treatments for ringworm.

Ringworm of the groin (*Tinea cruris*) presents as an itchy red area in the genital region and often spreads to the inside of the thighs. The problem is more common in men than in women and is commonly known as 'jock itch' in the USA. Treatment consists of topical antifungals; the use of powder formulations can be particularly valuable because they absorb perspiration.

Athlete's foot in practice

Case 1

Mark Roberts, the local plumber, is in his early twenties and captains the local football team on Sunday mornings. Today he wants to buy something for his athlete's foot, which he tells you he just can't get rid of. His girlfriend bought him some cream a few days ago but it doesn't seem to be having any effect. The skin between the third and fourth toes and between the second and third toes is affected. Mark tells you the skin is itchy and that 'it looks flaky'. He tells you that he has had athlete's foot before and that it keeps coming back again. He wears training shoes most of the time (he has them on now) and has used the cream his girlfriend bought 'most days'.

The pharmacist's view

From the answers he has given, it sounds as though Mark has athlete's foot. Once you have ascertained the identity of the cream he has been using, it might be appropriate to suggest the use of one of the imidazoles. Advice is also needed about foot hygiene and footwear and about regular use of treatment. If the problem has not cleared up after 2 weeks, Mark should see his doctor.

The doctor's view

With the correct advice from the pharmacist his problem should clear up. It sounds as if he expected the cream bought by his girlfriend to have been a rapid cure and it would be worthwhile explaining that with such infections he will have to persevere with treatment for much longer. A change in the type of footwear is also likely to be helpful.

Case 2

Linda Green asks if you can recommend anything for athlete's foot. She tells you that it affects her toes and the soles and top of her feet and is extremely itchy. When asked about the skin between her toes, she tells you she does not think the rash is between the toes. She says the skin is dry and red and has been like this for several days. Ms Green has not tried any medication to treat it.

The pharmacist's view

The symptoms which Linda Green has described do not sound like those of athlete's foot. The skin between the toes is not affected, so dermatitis is a possibility. Rather than recommend a product without being able to identity the cause of the problem, it would be better to refer Ms Green to her doctor.

The doctor's view

The description that the pharmacist has obtained does not sound like athlete's foot, which usually involves the cleft between the fourth and fifth toes. Referral to the doctor for diagnosis would be sensible.

Cold sores

Cold sores (herpes labialis) are caused by one of the most common viruses affecting humans worldwide. The virus responsible is the herpes simplex virus (HSV) of which there are two major types: HSV1 and HSV2. The former HSV1, typically causes infection around or in the mouth whereas the latter HSV2 is responsible for genital herpes infection. Occasionally, however, this situation is reversed with HSV2 affecting the face and HSV1 the genital area.

What you need to know
Age
Duration
Symptoms and appearance
Tingling
Pain
Location (current and previous)
Precipitating factors
Sunlight
Infection
Stress
Previous history
Medication

Significance of questions and answers

Age

Although initial infection, which is usually subclinical and goes unnoticed, occurs in childhood, cold sores are most commonly seen in adolescents and younger adults. Following the primary attack the virus is not completely eradicated and virus particles lie dormant in nerve roots until they are reactivated at a later stage. Although herpes infection is almost universal in childhood, not all those affected later experience cold sores and the reason for this is not fully understood. Recurrent cold sores occur in up to 25% of all adults and the frequency declines with age, although cold sores occur in patients of all ages. The incidence of cold sores is slightly higher in women than in men.

In an active primary herpes infection of childhood the typical picture is of a febrile child with a painful ulcerated mouth and enlarged lymph nodes. The herpetic lesions last for 3–6 days and can involve the outer skin surface as well as the inside of the mouth. Such patients should be referred to the doctor.

Duration

The duration of the symptoms is important as treatment with *acyclovir* is of most value if started early in the course of the infection (during the prodromal phase). Usually the infection is resolved within 1–2 weeks. Any lesions which have persisted longer need medical referral.

Symptoms and appearance

The symptoms of discomfort, tingling or irritation (prodromal phase) may occur in the skin for 2–3 days before the appearance of the cold sore. The cold sore starts with the development of minute blisters on top of inflamed, red, raised skin. The blisters may be filled with white matter. They quickly break down to produce a raw area with exudation and crusting by about the fourth day after their appearance. By around a week later, most lesions will have healed.

Cold sores are extremely painful and this is one of the critical diagnostic factors. Oral cancer can sometimes present a similar appearance to a cold sore. However, cancerous lesions are often painless and their long duration differentiates them from cold sores.

When a cold sore occurs for the first time it can be confused with a small patch of impetigo. Impetigo is usually more widespread, does not start with blisters and has a honey-coloured crust. Impetigo tends to spread out to form further patches and does not necessarily start close to the lips. It is less common than cold sores and tends to affect children. Since impetigo requires either topical or oral antibiotic treatment, the condition cannot be treated by the pharmacist.

If there is any doubt about the cause of the symptoms, the patient should be referred.

Location

Cold sores occur most often on the lips or face. Lesions inside the mouth or affecting the eye need medical referral.

Precipitating factors

It is known that cold sores can be precipitated by sunlight, wind, fever (during infections such as colds and flu), menstruation, being 'run down' and local trauma to the skin. Physical and emotional stress can also be triggers. Whilst it is often not possible to avoid these factors completely, the information is usually helpful for the sufferer.

Previous history

The fact that the cold sore is recurrent is helpful diagnostically. If a sore keeps on returning in the same place in a similar way then it is likely to be a cold sore. Most sufferers experience one to three attacks each year. Cold sores occur throughout the year, with a slightly increased incidence during the winter months. Information about the frequency and severity of the cold sore recurrence is helpful when recommending referral to the doctor, although the condition can usually be treated by the pharmacist.

In patients with atopic eczema, herpes infections can be severe and widespread. Such patients must be referred to their doctor.

Medication

It is helpful to enquire what creams and lotions have been used so far, what was used in previous episodes and what, if anything, helped last time.

Immunocompromised patients, for example those undergoing cytotoxic chemotherapy, are at risk of serious infection and should always be referred to their doctor.

When to refer
Babies and young children
Failure of an established sore to resolve
Severe or worsening sore
History of frequent cold sores
Sore lasting longer than 2 weeks
Painless sore
Patients with atopic eczema
Eye affected
Uncertain diagnosis
Immunocompromised patient

Management

Acyclovir

The most effective treatment is 5% *acyclovir cream*. This is an antiviral cream which accelerates healing, and is most effective if started as soon as symptoms first appear. *Acyclovir* is therefore a helpful recommendation for patients who suffer repeated attacks and know when a cold sore is going to appear. Such patients can be told that they should use treatment as soon as they feel the characteristic tingling or itching which precedes the appearance of a cold sore.

Acyclovir cream should be applied five times a day to the affected area. If healing is not complete, treatment can be continued for up to

5 more days, after which medical advice should be sought if the cold sore has not resolved. Some patients experience a transient stinging sensation after applying the cream. The affected skin may become dry and flaking in some cases.

Antiseptics

If the cold sore is well established an antibacterial topical treatment could be of some value in preventing a secondary infection. *Povidone-iodine 10%* in an alcoholic solution (antiseptic paint) also has an antiviral action and its alcoholic base helps to dry the sore. Other skin disinfection solutions such as *benzalkonium chloride* or *cetrimide* could also be used. *Povidone-iodine* should be avoided during pregnancy and when breast feeding. It is important to enquire whether or not there is a history of iodine sensitivity. Both *benzalkonium chloride* and *cetrimide* should be kept clear of contact with the eyes.

Bland creams

Keeping the cold sore moist will prevent drying and cracking which might predispose to secondary bacterial infection. For the patient who suffers only an occasional cold sore, a simple cream, perhaps containing an antiseptic agent, can help to reduce discomfort.

Practical points

Preventing cross-infection

Patients should be aware HSV1 is contagious and transmitted by direct contact. Tell patients to wash their hands after applying treatment to the cold sore. Women should be careful in applying eye make-up when they have a cold sore, to prevent infection affecting the eye. It is sensible not to share cutlery, towels, toothbrushes or face flannels until the cold sore has cleared up. Oral sex with someone who has a cold sore means a risk of genital herpes and should be avoided until the cold sore has gone.

Use of sunscreens

Sunscreen creams applied to and around the lips when patients are subject to increased sun exposure (e.g. during skiing and beach holidays) can be a useful preventive measure.

Stress

Sources of stresses in life could be looked at to see if changes are possible. It might be worthwhile recommending a discussion with the doctor about this.

Eczema herpeticum (Kaposi's varicelliform eruption)

Patients with atopic eczema are very susceptible to herpetic infection and show an abnormal response to the virus with widespread lesions and sometimes involvement of the central nervous system (CNS). These patients should avoid contact with anyone who has an active cold sore.

Warts and verrucae

Warts and verrucae are caused by a viral infection of the skin and have a high incidence in schoolchildren. Once immunity to the infecting virus is sufficiently high the lesions will disappear, but many patients and parents prefer active treatment for cosmetic reasons. Effective preparations are available over the counter (OTC), but correct use is essential if damage to surrounding skin is to be minimized.

What you need to know

Age
    Adult, child
Appearance and number of lesions
Location
Duration and history
Medication

Significance of questions and answers

Age

Warts can occur in children and adults: they are more common in children and peak incidence is found between the ages of 12 and 16 years. The peak incidence is thought to be due to higher exposure to the virus in schools and sports facilities. Warts and verrucae are both caused by the human papilloma virus, differing in their location.

Appearance

Warts appear as raised lesions with a roughened surface which are usually flesh coloured. Plantar warts occur on the weight-bearing areas of the sole and heel of the foot (verrucae). They have a different appearance from warts elsewhere on the body because the pressure from the body's weight pushes the lesion inwards, eventually producing pain when weight is applied during walking. Warts have a network of capillaries and, if pared, thrombosed, blackened capillaries or bleeding points will be seen. The presence of these capillaries provides a useful distinguishing feature between callouses and verrucae on the feet: if a corn or callous is pared, no such dark points will be seen; instead layers of white keratin will be present. The thrombosed capillaries are sometimes thought, incorrectly, to be the 'root' of the verruca by the patient. The pharmacist can correct this misconception when explaining the purpose and method of treatment (discussed later in this section).

Multiple warts

Warts may occur singly, or as several lesions. Molluscum contagiosum is a condition in which the lesions may resemble warts and where another type of viral infection is the cause. Closer examination shows that the lesions contain a central plug of material (consisting of viral particles) which can be removed by squeezing. The location of molluscum contagiosum tends to differ from that of warts—the eyelids, face, armpits and trunk may be involved. Such cases are best referred to the doctor, since self-treatment would be inappropriate.

Location

The palms or backs of the hands are common sites for warts, as is the area around the fingernails. People who bite or pick their nails are more susceptible to warts around them. Warts sometimes occur on the face and referral to the doctor is the best option in such cases. Since treatment with OTC products is destructive in nature, self-treatment of facial warts can lead to scarring and should never be attempted.

Parts of the skin which are subject to regular trauma or friction are more likely to be affected, since damage to the skin facilitates entry of the virus. Plantar warts (verrucae) are found on the sole of the foot and may be present singly or as several lesions.

Anogenital

Anogenital warts are caused by a different type of the human papilloma virus and require medical referral for examination, diagnosis and treatment.

Duration and history

It is known that most warts will disappear spontaneously within a time period of between 6 months and 2 years. The younger the patient, the more quickly the lesions are likely to remit.

Any change in the appearance of a wart should be treated with suspicion and referral to the doctor advised. Skin cancers are sometimes mistakenly thought to be warts by patients, and the pharmacist can establish how long the lesion has been present and any changes which have occurred. Signs which are related to skin cancer are described in *Practical points* below.

Medication

Diabetic patients should not use OTC products to treat warts or verrucae since impaired circulation can lead to delayed healing, ulceration or even gangrene. Peripheral neuropathy may mean that even extensive damage to the skin may not provoke a sensation of pain.

Warts can be a major problem if the immune system is suppressed by either disease (e.g. human immunodeficiency virus (HIV) infection; lymphoma) or drugs (e.g. cyclosporin to prevent rejection of a transplant).

The pharmacist should ask whether any treatment has been attempted already and if so, its identity and the method of use. Commonly, treatments are not used for a sufficiently long period of time because patients' expectations are often of a fast 'cure'.

When to refer

Changed appearance of lesions: size, colour
Bleeding
Itching
Genital warts
Facial warts
Immunocompromised patients

Treatment timescale

Treatment with OTC preparations should produce a successful outcome within 3 months; if not, referral is necessary.

Management

Treatment of warts and verrucae aims to reduce the size of the lesion by gradual destruction of the skin. Continous application of the selected preparation for several weeks or months may be needed and it is important to explain this to the patient if compliance with treatment is to be achieved. Surrounding healthy skin should be protected during treatment (see *Practical points* below).

Salicylic acid

Salicylic acid may be considered to be the treatment of choice for warts; it acts by softening and destroying the skin, thus mechanically removing infected tissue. Preparations are available in a variety of strengths, sometimes in collodion-type bases which help retain the *salicylic acid* in contact with the wart. Ointments, gels and plasters provide a selection of methods of application. Preparations should be kept well away from the eyes and applied using an orange stick or other applicator, not with the fingers.

Podophyllum

Podophyllum has a cytotoxic (antimitotic) action, preventing cell division. Its main uses are in verrucae and anogenital warts. As it is strongly irritant both to the skin and to mucous membranes, care must be taken to ensure that application is restricted to the wart itself. Application of preparations containing *podophyllum* to the wart twice weekly will be sufficient.

Pregnancy

Pregnant women should not use preparations containing *podophyllum* because of the risk of damage to the fetus which may occur following absorption of *podophyllum*. The toxicity of *podophyllum* means that adverse systemic effects have been reported after topical use. However, the risk of such effects is low providing the area of the skin treated is small.

Formaldehyde

Formaldehyde is used for the treatment of verrucae; it is considered to be less suitable for warts on the hands because of its irritant effect on the skin. The thicker skin layer on the sole of the feet protects against this irritant action. A gel formulation is available for the treatment of verrucae and is applied twice a day. *Formalin soaks* are sometimes used for verrucae and it is important to tell the patient to protect the unaffected skin, particularly between the toes, with *white soft paraffin* as otherwise cracking and soreness will result. The foot is soaked for 10 minutes each day. Both *formaldehyde* and *glutaraldehyde* have an unpredictable action and are not first-line treatments for warts, though they may be useful in resistant cases.

Glutaraldehyde

Glutaraldehyde is used in a 5 or 10% gel or solution to treat warts; it is not used for anogenital warts and is generally used for verrucae. Its effect on viruses is variable. Patients should be warned that *glutaraldehyde* will stain the skin brown although this will fade after treatment has stopped.

Practical points

Application of treatments

Treatments containing *salicylic acid* should be applied daily. The treatment is helped by prior soaking of the affected hand or foot in warm water for 5–10 minutes to soften and hydrate the skin, increasing the action of the *salicylic acid*. Removal of dead skin from the surface of the wart by gentle rubbing with a pumice stone or emery board ensures that the next application reaches the surface of the lesion. Occlusion of the wart using an adhesive plaster helps to keep the skin macerated, maximizing the effectiveness of *salicylic acid*.

Protection. Protection of the surrounding skin is important and can be achieved by applying a layer of *petroleum jelly* to prevent the treatment from making contact with healthy skin. Application of the liquid or gel using an orange stick will help to confine the substance to the lesion itself.

Warts and skin cancer

Premalignant and malignant lesions can sometimes be thought to be warts by the patient. There are different types of skin cancer. They can be divided into two categories: those not pigmented (i.e. skin coloured), and those pigmented (i.e. brown).

Non-pigmented. In this first group, which is more likely to occur in the elderly, the signs might include a persisting small ulcer or sore which slowly enlarges but never seems to heal. Sometimes a crust forms but when it falls off the lesion is still present. In the case of a basal cell carcinoma (rodent ulcer) the lesion typically has a circular, raised and rolled edge.

Pigmented. Pigmented lesions or moles can turn malignant. These can occur in patients of a much younger age than the first group. Changes in nature or appearance of pigmented skin lesions which warrant referral for further investigation include:
   increase in size
   irregular, wavy outline
   colour change, especially to black
   itching or bleeding.

Length of treatment required

Several weeks' continuous treatment is usually needed—up to 3 months for both warts and verrucae. Patients need to know that a long period of treatment will be required and that they should not expect instant or rapid success. An invitation to come back to see the pharmacist and report progress can help the pharmacist to monitor the treatment. If treatment has not been successful after 3 months, referral for removal using liquid nitrogen may be required.

Verrucae and swimming pools

Viruses are able to penetrate moist skin more easily than dry skin and it has been suggested that the high level of use of swimming pools has contributed to the high incidence of verrucae. Theoretically walking barefoot on abrasive surfaces by the pool or changing area can lead to infected material from the verruca being rubbed into the flooring. There has been controversy about whether the wearing of protective rubber socks can protect against the spread of verrucae. Also the wearing of this conspicuous article might in itself create stigma for the child involved.

Scabies

Infestation by the scabies mite, *Sarcoptes scabei*, causes a character-istically intense itching, which is worse during the night. The itch of scabies can be severe and scratching of the skin can lead to changes in the appearance of the skin. It is therefore necessary to take a careful history. Scabies goes through peaks and troughs of prevalence and pharmacists need to be aware when a peak is occurring.

What you need to know
Age
Infant, child, adult
Symptoms
Itching, rash
Presence of burrows
History
Signs of infection
Medication

Significance of questions and answers

Age

Scabies infestation can occur at any age, from infancy onwards. The pharmacist may feel it best to refer infants and young children to the doctor if scabies is suspected.

Symptoms

The scabies mite burrows down into the skin and lives under the surface of the skin. The presence of the mites sets up an allergic reaction, thought to be due to the insect's coat and exudates, resulting in intense itching. A characteristic feature of scabies is that itching is worse at night and can lead to loss of sleep.

Burrows can sometimes be seen as small thread-like grey lines. The lines are raised, wavy and about 5–10 mm long. Commonly infested sites include the web space of the fingers and toes, wrists, armpits, buttocks and genital area. Patients may have a rash which does not always correspond to the areas of infestation. The rash may be patchy and diffuse or dense and erythematous. It is more commonly found around the midriff, underarms, buttocks, inside the thighs and around the ankles.

In adults, scabies rarely affects the scalp and face, but in infants aged 2 years or under and in the elderly, involvement of the head is more common, especially the postauricular fold.

Burrows may be indistinct or may have been disguised by scratching which has broken and excoriated the skin. Scabies can mimic other skin conditions and may not present with the 'classic' features. The itch tends to be generalized rather than in specific areas. In immuno-compromised or debilitated patients (e.g. the elderly), scabies presents differently. The affected skin can become thickened and crusted. Mites survive under the crust and any sections which become dislodged are infectious to others because of the living mites they contain.

History

The itch of scabies can take several (6–8) weeks to develop in someone who has not been infested previously. The scabies mite is transmitted by close personal contact, so patients can be asked whether anyone else they know is affected by the same symptoms, for example other family members, boyfriends and girlfriends.

Signs of infection

Scratching can lead to excoriation, so that secondary infections such as impetigo can occur. The presence of a weeping yellow discharge or yellow crusts would be indications for referral to the doctor for treatment.

Medication

It is important for the pharmacist to establish whether any treatment has been tried already and, if so, its identity. The patient should be asked about how any treatment has been used, since incorrect use can result in treatment failure. The itch of scabies may continue for several days or even weeks after successful treatment, so the fact that itching has not subsided does not necessarily mean that treatment has been unsuccessful.

When to refer

Babies and children
Infected skin
Treatment failure
Unclear diagnosis

Management

Malathion lotion and *permethrin cream* are effective scabicides (acaricides) and are the preferred treatments. Aqueous lotions are used in preference to alcoholic versions because the latter sting and irritate excoriated skin. All scabicides can themselves cause irritation of the skin and this should be explained to patients, who may otherwise think the treatment has been ineffective and that their condition has become worse. *Benzyl benzoate* application is rarely used these days because of its particularly irritant effect. *Lindane* and *Monosulfiram lotion* are no longer available. Medical supervision is required for the treatment of scabies in children aged under 2 years.

The treatment is applied to the entire body, from the neck downwards but not the neck, face and scalp in adults. However, in children aged under 2 years and the elderly the advice now is to include the scalp, neck, face (avoiding eyes and mouth) and ears in the application unless the product packaging contra-indicates this. This recommendation is because treatment failure has occurred because the head, neck and scalp were not treated.

Patients are sometimes unsure about how to apply the lotion they have been told to use and simple advice is that they should pour the preparation into a bowl, then apply it using a clean, broad paintbrush, cotton wool or a shaving brush. Patients should be told to apply the preparation to the whole body, not just to the areas where burrows have been found. Particular attention should be paid to the webs of fingers, toes, to the soles of the feet and to brushing lotion under the ends of the fingernails and toenails. Providing the treatment is applied properly, a second application of *malathion* or *permethrin* is not necessary. If *benzyl benzoate* is used, up to three applications on consecutive days may be needed. Traditionally patients have been told to have a hot bath before applying the scabicide but this is no longer recommended (see below).

Malathion

Malathion is effective for the treatment of scabies and pediculosis (head lice). For one application in an adult 100 ml of lotion should be sufficient. The aqueous lotion should be used in scabies. The lotion is applied over the whole body—omitting the head and neck in adults (unless elderly) and children over 2 years old—and left on for 24 hours, without bathing, after which it is washed off. If the hands are washed with soap and water during the 24 hours, *malathion* should be reapplied to the hands. Skin irritation may sometimes occur.

Permethrin

The cream formulation is used in the treatment of scabies. For a single application in an adult 30–60 g of cream (1–2 tubes) is needed. The cream is applied to the whole body and left on for a minimum of 8 hours, preferably for 24 hours, before being washed off. If the hands are washed with soap and water within 8 hours of application, another application of cream should be made to the hands. *Permethrin* can be used for children aged from 2 months upwards; medical supervision is required for its use in children aged under 2 years and in elderly patients (aged 70 and over). *Permethrin* can itself cause itching and reddening of the skin.

Benzyl benzoate application

This preparation is a 25% strength application, which is used solely in the treatment of scabies.

Irritant nature

Benzyl benzoate itself is irritant in nature and can cause stinging, itching and burning of the skin as well as occasional skin rashes. For this reason, it is not recommended for babies or children and should not be used for patients with eczema or with scratched and broken skin, in whom severe stinging may occur.

Application

The preparation should be applied to the whole body except the head and neck and left to dry on the skin. A second application should be made the next day, without bathing or washing off the first. The second application is washed off 24 hours later. *Benzyl benzoate* is extremely irritant to the eyes and mucous membranes; it should be kept well away from the eyes.

Practical points

1 The itch will continue and may become worse in the first few days after treatment. The reason for this is thought to be the release of allergen from dead mites. Patients need to be told that the itch will not stop straight away after treatment. *Crotamiton cream* or lotion could be used to relieve the symptoms providing the skin is not badly excoriated. *Calamine cream* is another treatment option and an oral antihistamine such as *promethazine* may be considered if the itch is severe.

2 Good advice would be to apply the treatment immediately before bedtime (leaving time for it to dry). Because the hands are likely to be affected by scabies it is important not to wash the hands after application of the treatment and to reapply the preparation if the hands are washed within the treatment period.

3 Patients with scabies were traditionally advised to have a hot bath before applying their treatment. The theory was that a hot bath would open up the mites' burrows, making it easier for the scabicide to reach the mites. This advice is no longer recommended: there is no evidence that a hot bath increases the effectiveness of scabicides but there is a real possibility that increased absorption of the scabicide could occur through warm, hydrated skin, removing the active substance from its site of action on the skin's surface.

4 All members of the family or household should be treated, preferably on the same day. Because the itch of scabies may take several weeks to develop, people may be infested but symptomless. It is thought that patients may not develop symptoms for up to 8 weeks after infestation. The incubation period of the scabies mite is 3 weeks, so reinfestation may occur from other family or household members.

5 The scabies mite can only live for around a day after leaving its host and transmission is almost always caused by close personal contact. It is unlikely that infestation could occur from bedclothes or clothing. After treatment for scabies, bedclothes and clothing should be washed, but there is no need for disinfection.

6 Other possible infestations include those caused by pet fleas and bed bugs. Pet fleas are common and patients may present with small reddened swellings, often on the lower legs and around the ankles where the pet has come into contact with the skin. Questioning may reveal that a pet cat or dog has recently been acquired or that a pet has not been treated with insecticide for some time. Regular checks for fleas and use of insecticides will prevent the problem occurring in the future. A range of proprietary products is available to treat either the pet or bedding and carpets. A second treatment should be applied 2 weeks after the first to eradicate any fleas which have hatched since the first application.

Pet flea bites can be treated with *topical hydrocortisone* in anyone over 10 years old. Alternatively, an antipruritic such as *crotamiton* (with or without *hydrocortisone*) or *aqueous calamine cream* can be recommended.

Dandruff

Dandruff is a chronic relapsing condition of the scalp which responds to treatment but returns when treatment is stopped. The condition usually appears during puberty and reaches a peak in early adulthood. Dandruff has been estimated to affect one in two people aged between 20 and 30 and up to four in 10 of those aged between 30 and 40. The condition is associated with the yeast *Pityrosporum ovale*, as is seborrhoeic dermatitis. Diagnosis is straightforward and effective treatments are available over the counter (OTC).

What you need to know

Appearance
    Presence of scales
    Colour and texture of scales
Location
    Scalp
    Eyebrows; paranasal clefts
    Others
Severity
Previous history
    Psoriasis
    Seborrhoeic dermatitis
Aggravating factors
Medication

Significance of questions and answers

Appearance

Dandruff is characterised by greyish-white flakes or scales on the scalp and an itchy scalp as a result of excessive scaling. In dandruff the epidermal cell turnover is at twice the rate of those without the condition. The differential diagnosis for severe dandruff would consider seborrhoeic dermatitis and psoriasis. In the latter conditions both the appearance and location would be different.

In seborrhoeic dermatitis the scales are yellowish and greasy-looking and there is usually some inflammation with reddening and crusting of the affected skin.

In psoriasis the scales are silvery-white and associated with red, patchy plaques and inflammation.

So inflammation and redness of the scalp are absent in dandruff but present in seborrhoeic dermatitis and psoriasis.

Location

In dandruff the scalp is the only area affected. Seborrhoeic dermatitis affects the areas where there is greatest sebaceous gland activity so it usually involves other areas. The eyebrows, eyelashes, moustache, paranasal clefts, behind the ears, nape of neck, forehead and chest may be affected.

In infants seborrhoeic dermatitis is common and occurs as cradle cap, appearing in the first 12 weeks of life.

Psoriasis can affect the scalp but other areas are involved. The knees and elbows are commonly involved but the face is rarely affected. This latter point distinguishes psoriasis from seborrhoeic dermatitis, where the face is often affected.

Severity

Dandruff is generally a mild condition. However, the itching scalp may lead to scratching, which may break the skin, causing soreness and the possibility of infection. If the scalp is very sore or there are signs of infection (crusting or weeping) referral should be indicated.

Previous history

Since dandruff is a chronic relapsing condition there will usually be a previous history of fluctuating symptoms. There is a seasonal variation in symptoms, which generally improve in summer in response to UVB light. *Pityrosporum ovale* is unaffected by UVA light.

Aggravating factors

Hair dyes and perms can irritate the scalp. Inadequate rinsing after shampooing the hair can leave traces of shampoo causing irritation and itching.

Stress can exacerbate seborrhoeic dermatitis and psoriasis whereas dandruff is a stable condition.

Psoriasis can be exacerbated by drugs (e.g. *chloroquine*).

Medication

Various treatments may already have been tried. It is important to identify what has been tried and how it was used. Dandruff treatments need to be applied to the scalp and to be left for at least 5 minutes for best effect. However, if an appropriate treatment has been correctly used with no improvement, referral should be considered.

When to refer

Suspected psoriasis
Signs of infection
Unresponsive to appropriate treatment

Treatment timescale

Dandruff should start to improve within 1–2 weeks of beginning treatment.

Management

The aim of treatment is to reduce the level of *Pityrosporum ovale* on the scalp so agents with antifungal action are effective. *Ketoconazole, selenium sulphide, zinc pyrithione* and *coal tar* are effective. The results from studies suggest that *ketoconazole* is the most and *coal tar* is the least effective. All treatments need to be left on the scalp for 3–5 minutes for full effect.

Ketoconazole

Transferred from prescription only medicine (POM) to pharmacy medicine (P) in 1996, *ketoconazole* is extremely effective in the treatment of dandruff. The formulation available is *ketoconazole 2% shampoo*. The treatment should be used twice a week for 2–4 weeks after which usage should reduce to weekly or fortnightly as needed to prevent recurrence.

The shampoo can also be used in seborrhoeic dermatitis. Whilst shampooing the lather can be applied to the other affected areas and left before rinsing.

Ketoconazole is not absorbed through the scalp and side effects are extremely rare. There have been occasional reports of allergic reactions.

Selenium sulphide 2.5%

Selenium sulphide has been shown to be effective and works by reducing the cell turnover rate (cytostatic effect). The shampoos containing this ingredient are P products. Twice-weekly use for the first 2 weeks is followed by weekly use for the next 2 weeks; it then can be used as needed. The hair and scalp should be thoroughly rinsed after using *selenium sulphide shampoo*, otherwise discoloration of blonde, grey or dyed hair can result. Frequent use can make the scalp greasy and can therefore exacerbate seborrhoeic dermatitis. Products containing selenium sulphide should not be used within 48 hours of colouring or perming the hair. Contact dermatitis has occasionally been reported. Selenium sulphide should not be applied to inflamed or broken skin.

Zinc pyrithione

Shampoos containing this ingredient are general sales list (GSL) products and are generally considered cosmetic products. *Zinc pyrithione* is effective against dandruff and has a cytostatic effect. It should be used twice weekly for the first 2 weeks and then once weekly as required.

Coal tar

Findings from research studies indicate that this is the least effective of the anti-dandruff agents. Modern formulations are pleasanter than the traditional ones but some people still find the smell of *coal tar* unacceptable. *Coal tar* can cause skin sensitization and is a photosensitizer.

Practical points

Continuing treatment

Patients need to understand that the treatment will not cure their dandruff permanently and that it will be sensible to use the treatment on a less frequent basis to prevent their dandruff coming back.

Treating the scalp

It is the scalp that needs to be treated rather than the hair. The treatment should be applied to the scalp and massaged gently.

All products need to be left on the scalp for 5 minutes before rinsing for the full effect to be gained.

Standard shampoos

There is debate amongst experts as to whether dandruff is caused by infrequent hair washing. However, it is generally agreed that frequent washing (at least three times a week) is an important part of managing dandruff. Between applications of their treatment the patient can continue to use their normal shampoo. Some may wish to wash their hair with their normal shampoo before using the dandruff treatment shampoo.

Hair products

Gel, mousse and hairspray can still be used and will not adversely affect treatment for dandruff.

Hair loss

The two major causes of hair loss are alopecia androgenetica (male pattern baldness, sometimes known as common baldness because it can affect women) and alopecia areata. The first of these may be treatable, but there are currently no treatments which the pharmacy can offer for alopecia areata. Although hair loss has been regarded largely as a cosmetic problem, the psychological effects on sufferers can be substantial. A sympathetic approach is therefore essential. Occasionally hair loss may be associated with certain medical conditions such as myxoedema (underactive thyroid).

What you need to know
Male or female
History and duration of hair loss
Location and size of affected areas
Other symptoms
Influencing factors
Medication

Significance of questions and answers

Male or female
Men and women may both suffer from alopecia androgenetica or alopecia areata. Alopecia areata can affect people at any age.

History and duration of hair loss
Alopecia androgenetica is characterised by gradual onset. In men the pattern of loss is recession of the hair line at the front and/or loss of hair on the top of the scalp. In women the hair loss is generalized and there is an increase in the parting width. Another pattern of hair loss in women in the 20 plus age group is increased shedding of hair but without any increase in the parting width. This latter pattern is not due to alopecia androgenetica and it is thought that the cause may be nutritional. Hair loss in women is increasingly recognized as a problem.

Alopecia areata may be sudden and result in patchy hair loss. The cause of alopecia areata remains unknown but it is thought that the problem may be autoimmune in origin.

Location and size of affected area

If the affected area is less than 10 cm in diameter in alopecia androgenetica then treatment may be worth trying.

Other symptoms

Coarsening of the hair and hair loss can occur as a result of hypothyroidism (myxoedema) where other symptoms might include a feeling of tiredness or being 'run down' and a deepening of the voice.

Inflammatory conditions of the scalp such as ringworm infection (*Tinea capitis*) can cause hair loss. Other symptoms here would be itching and redness of the scalp with an advancing reddened edge of the infected area. Referral would be needed in such cases.

Influencing factors

Hormonal changes during and after pregnancy mean that hair loss is common both during pregnancy and after the baby has been born. While this is often distressing for the woman concerned it is completely normal and she can be reassured that the hair will grow back. Treatment is not appropriate.

Medication

Cytotoxic drugs are well known for causing hair loss. Anticoagulants, lipid-lowering agents and vitamin A (in overdose) have also been associated with hair loss. Such cases should be referred to the doctor.

When to refer

Alopecia areata
Suspected drug-induced hair loss
Suspected hypothyroidism

Treatment timescale

Treatment with *minoxidil* may take up to four months to show full effect.

Management

Minoxidil

The only treatment licensed for use in hair loss is *minoxidil*, available as a 2% lotion with the drug dissolved in an aqueous alcohol solution. Propylene glycol is included to enhance absorption. The mechanism of action of *minoxidil* in baldness is unknown. The earlier *minoxidil* is used in balding, the more likely it is to be successful. Treatment is most likely to work where the bald area is less than 10 cm in diameter, where there is still some hair present and the person has been losing hair for less than 10 years. The manufacturers of *minoxidil* say that the product works best in men with hair loss or thinning at the top of the scalp and in women in a generalized thinning over the whole scalp, both manifestations of alopecia androgenetica. Up to one in three users in such circumstances report hair regrowth of non-vellus (normal) hair and stabilization of hair loss. A further one in three are likely to report some growth of vellus (fine, downy) hair. The final third will not see any improvement.

It is important that patients understand the factors that make successful treatment more or less likely and that their expectations are realistic. Some patients may still want to try the treatment, even where the chances of improvement are small.

After 4–6 weeks the patient can expect to see a reduction in hair loss. It will take 4 months for any hair regrowth to be seen and some dermatologists suggest continuing use for a year before abandoning treatment. Initially the new hair will be soft and downy but it should gradually thicken to become like normal hair in texture and appearance.

Application

The lotion should be applied twice daily to the dry scalp and lightly massaged into the affected area of the scalp. The hair should be clean and dry and the lotion should be left to dry naturally. The hair should not be washed for at least an hour after using the lotion.

Caution

Irritant and allergic reactions to the alcohol/propylene glycol vehicle sometimes occur. A small amount (approximately 1.5%) of the drug is absorbed systemically and there is the theoretical possibility of a hypotensive effect but this appears to be unlikely in practice. *Minoxidil* is also known to cause a reflex increase in heart rate. While this is a theoretical risk where such small amounts of the drug are involved tachycardia and palpitations have occasionally been reported. The manufacturers advise against use in anyone with hypertension, angina or heart disease without first checking with the patient's doctor. Although no specific problems have been reported the manufacturers advise against use when pregnant or breastfeeding.

It is important to explain to patients that they will need to make a long-term commitment to the treatment should it be successful. Treatment must be continued indefinitely: new hair growth will fall out 2–3 months after treatment is stopped. A year's treatment currently costs about £380.

Minoxidil should not be used in alopecia areata or in hair loss related to pregnancy.

Psoriasis

People with this skin condition usually present to the doctor rather than the pharmacist. At the time of first presentation the doctor is the most appropriate first line of help and pharmacists should always refer cases of suspected but undiagnosed psoriasis. The diagnosis is not always easy and needs confirming. In the situation of a confirmed diagnosis in a relatively chronic situation, the pharmacist can offer continuation of the treatment where the products are available over the counter (OTC).

This is a condition where continued management and monitoring by the pharmacist is reasonable, with referral back to the doctor when there is an exacerbation or for periodic review. Jointly agreed guidelines between pharmacist and doctors are valuable here.

Psoriasis occurs worldwide with variation in incidence between different ethnic groups. The incidence for white Europeans is about 2%. Although there is a genetic influence, environmental factors are thought to be important.

What you need to know
Appearance
Psychological factors
Diagnosis

Significance of questions and answers

Appearance
In its most common form there are raised large red scaly patches/plaques over the extensor surfaces of the elbow and knee. The patches are symmetrical and sometimes there is a patch present over the lower back area. The scalp is often involved.

Psychological factors
In some people these patches are very long standing and show little change. With other people the skin changes worsen and spread to other parts of the body, often in response to a stressful event. This is particularly distressing for the person involved who then has to cope with the stress of having a relapse of psoriasis as well as the precipitating event.

The psychological impact of having a chronic skin disorder such as psoriasis must not be underestimated. There is still a significant stigma connected with skin disease. There can be a mistaken belief that the rash is contagious. There is a cultural pressure to have a 'perfect' body as defined by the fashion industry and media. Psoriasis can understandably cause loss of self esteem, embarrassment and depression. This is further compounded by the fact that there is no cure for psoriasis, although treatment will usually result in remission to some extent. There are various creams and ointments available but many of these are messy, smelly, stain clothes and are time-consuming to apply. The treatments do not always work, can cause sore skin and stain normal skin around the psoriatic plaque. The prospect of spending an hour before going to bed applying creams, clearing up the skin scales from the floor and getting into bed with smelly ointments is not an attractive one.

Diagnosis

The diagnosis of psoriasis can be confusing. In the typical situation described above it is straightforward. In addition to affecting the extensor surfaces, psoriasis can typically involve the scalp (also see p. 167). Often the fingernails shows signs of pitting which is a useful diagnostic guide. However, psoriasis can present with differing patterns which can be confused with other skin disorders. In guttate psoriasis a widespread rash of small scaly patches develops quickly affecting large areas of the body. This most typically occurs in children or young adults and may be triggered by a streptococcal sore throat. In general practice the most common differential diagnosis to guttate psoriasis is pityriasis rosea. This latter condition is a self-limiting one which usually settles down within 8 weeks.

Psoriasis can also involve the flexural surfaces, the groin area, palms, soles, and nails. The most common alternative diagnostic possibilities in these situations include eczema or fungal infections.

In 7% of people who have psoriasis there is an associated arthritis which usually affects a single joint but can be more severe and identical to rheumatoid arthritis.

Management

This is dependent on many factors, for example, nature and severity of psoriasis, understanding the aims of the treatment, ability to apply creams, and whether the person is pregnant (some treatments are teratogenic). As always, it is particularly important for the doctor to deal with the person's ideas, concerns and expectations, to appreciate how that person's life is affected by the condition, to give a relevant, understandable explanation and to mutually agree whether to treat or not, and, if so, how.

Topical treatments (e.g. *unguentum Merck, cetomacrogol, emulsifying ointment, yellow soft paraffin wax*)

The doctor is likely to offer a topical treatment. The possibilities include recommending an emollient, for example, *unguentum Merck, cetomacrogol, emulsifying ointment* or *yellow soft paraffin wax*. These can be used alone or in conjunction with active *dithranol* therapy. In the past this was traditionally made up in *Lassar's paste* which was effective but messy, with staining and local irritation. The newer proprietary creams (0.1–2%) are more acceptable especially when used for one short contact (30 minute) period each day and removed using an emollient. Some people are very sensitive to *dithranol* as it can cause quite severe skin irritation. It is usual to start with the lowest concentration and build up slowly to the strongest concentration that can be tolerated. Users should wash their hands after application. It should not be applied to the face, flexures or genitalia. There are some people who are unable to tolerate it at all.

Calcipotriol or tacalcitol

A newer topical treatment includes a vitamin D derivative available as *calcipotriol* or *tacalcitol*. This does not smell or stain and has been widely used in the treatment of mild to moderate psoriasis. It appears that it is as beneficial in efficacy as *dithranol*. If overused there is a risk of causing hypercalcaemia. It is now available as a scalp application as well as an ointment.

Topical steroids

Topical steroids should generally be restricted to use in the flexures or on the scalp. Although effective in suppressing skin plaques on the body, large amounts are required over time as the condition is a chronic one, resulting in severe steroid side effects.

Second line treatment

Referral by a doctor to a dermatologist may be necessary when there is diagnostic uncertainty, when the doctor's treatment fails, or in severe cases. Second line treatment may include phototherapy or systemic therapy with *methotrexate, etretinate* or *cyclosporin*. Unfortunately all of these have potentially serious side effects.

Painful Conditions

Headache

The most common types of headache which the community pharmacist is likely to encounter are tension headache, migraine and sinusitis. Careful questioning can distinguish causes which are potentially more serious so that referral to the doctor can be advised.

Significance of questions and answers

Age

The pharmacist would be well advised to refer any child with a headache to the doctor, especially if there is an associated history of injury or trauma to the head, for example from a fall. Children with severe pain across the back of the head and neck rigidity should be referred immediately. Elderly patients sometimes suffer a headache a few days after a fall involving a bang to the head. Such cases may be the result of a slow bleed into the brain causing a subdural haematoma and require immediate referral.

Duration

Any headache which lasts for longer than a few hours requires referral.

Nature and site of pain

Traditionally, a tension (psychogenic) headache has been described as a dull ache, while the headache of a migraine has been described as a pounding or throbbing pain. However, the nature of the pain alone is not sufficient evidence on which to decide whether the headache is likely to be from a minor or more serious cause.

A steady, dull pain which feels deep-sited, is severe, and is aggravated by lying down requires referral, since it may be due to raised intracranial pressure from a brain tumour, infection or other cause.

Classical migraine is unilateral, affecting one side of the head, especially over the forehead. A tension headache may be described as a weight pressing on top of the head, a band across the forehead, around the head or at the back of the head and neck.

Rarely, a sudden severe pain which develops at the back of the head may signify a subarachnoid haemorrhage. Sufferers may describe the onset of the pain like being struck on the back of the head with a brick. It occurs when a small blood vessel at the base of the brain leaks blood into the cerebrospinal fluid surrounding the brain. It may be associated with raised blood pressure. Urgent medical referral is essential.

Frequency and timing of symptoms

Pharmacists should regard a headache which is worse in the morning and which improves during the day as particularly serious, since this may be a sign of raised intracranial pressure.

Previous history

It is always reassuring to know that the headache experienced is the usual type for that person. In other words it has similar characteristics in nature and site but not necessarily in severity to headaches experienced over previous years. This fact makes it much less likely to be from a serious cause, whereas new or different headaches (especially in people aged over 45) may be a warning sign of a more serious condition. Migraine sufferers typically suffer from recurrent episodes of their headaches. In some cases the headaches occur in clusters. The pain may be present daily for 2–3 weeks and then be absent for months or years.

Associated symptoms

Children with unsteadiness and clumsiness associated with a headache should be referred.

Classical migraine

Classical migraine is often associated with alterations in vision before an attack starts, the so-called prodromal phase. Patients may describe seeing flashing lights or zigzag lines. During the prodromal phase, patients may experience tingling or numbness on one side of the body, in the lips, fingers, face or hands. Migraines are also associated with nausea and sometimes vomiting. Patients often get relief from lying in a darkened room and say that bright light hurts their eyes during an attack of migraine. Classical migraine is three times more common in women than in men.

Common migraine

There are other forms of migraine which do not fit the classical description above. In common migraine there is no prodromal phase, both sides of the head may be affected and gastrointestinal (GI) symptoms such as nausea and vomiting may occur. Cluster headaches involve, as their name suggests, a number of headaches one after the other. The pain can be excruciating and attacks can be days, weeks or months apart. A cluster headache is often accompanied by a painful, watering eye.

Sinusitis

Sinusitis may complicate a respiratory viral infection (e.g. cold) or allergy such as hay fever which causes inflammation and swelling of the mucosal lining of the sinuses. The increased mucus produced within the sinus cannot drain, a secondary bacterial infection develops and the pressure builds up, causing pain. The pain is felt behind and around the eye and usually only one side is affected. The headache may be associated with rhinorrhoea or nasal congestion. The affected sinus often feels tender when pressure is applied. It is typically worse on bending forwards or lying down.

Temporal arteritis

In temporal arteritis, which usually occurs in older patients, the arteries which run through the temples become inflamed. They may appear red and are painful and thickened to the touch. However, these signs are not always present. Any elderly patient presenting with a severe frontal or temporal headache which persists and is associated with a general feeling of being unwell should be referred immediately. Temporal arteritis is a curable disease and delay in diagnosis and treatment may lead to blindness. This is because the blood vessels to the eyes are also affected by inflammation. Treatment usually involves high-dose steroids and is successful providing the diagnosis is made sufficiently early.

Precipitating factors

Tension (psychogenic) headache may be precipitated by stress, for example pressure at work, or a family argument. Certain foods have been reported to precipitate migraine attacks, for example chocolate and cheese. Migraine headaches may also be triggered by emotional and psychological factors or by hormonal changes. In women, migraine attacks may be associated with the menstrual cycle.

Recent trauma or injury

Any patient presenting with a headache who has had a recent head injury or trauma to the head should be referred to the doctor immediately because bruising or haemorrhage may occur, causing a rise in intracranial pressure. The pharmacist should look out for drowsiness or any sign of impaired consciousness. Persistent vomiting after the injury is also a sign of raised intracranial pressure.

Recent eye test

Headaches associated with periods of reading, writing or other close work may be due to deteriorating eyesight and a sight test may be worth recommending to see whether spectacles are needed.

Medication

The nature of any prescribed medication should be established, since the headache might be a side effect of medication, for example nitrates used in the treatment of angina.

Contraceptive pill

Any woman taking the combined oral contraceptive pill and reporting migraine-type headaches, either for the first time or as an exacerbation of existing migraine, should be referred to the doctor, since this may be an early warming of cerebrovascular changes.

Occasionally, a headache is caused by hypertension but, contrary to popular opinion, such headaches are not common and only occur when the blood pressure is extremely high. Nevertheless, the pharmacist should consider the patient's medication carefully. In drug interactions which have led to a rise in blood pressure, for example between a sympatho-mimetic such as *phenylpropanolamine* and a monoamine oxidase inhibitor, a headache is likely to occur as a symptom.

The patient may already be taking a non-steroidal anti-inflammatory drug (NSAID) or other analgesic on prescription and duplication of treatments should be avoided, since toxicity may result.

If over-the-counter (OTC) treatment has already been tried without improvement, referral is advisable.

Treatment timescale

If the headache does not respond to OTC analgesics within a day, referral is advisable.

Management

The pharmacist's choice of oral analgesic is limited to three main agents: *aspirin, paracetamol* and *ibuprofen*. These are often combined with other constituents such as *codeine, dihydrocodeine, doxylamine* and *caffeine*. Over-the-counter analgesics are available in a variety of dosage forms and, in addition to traditional tablets and capsules, syrups, soluble tablets and sustained release dosage forms are available for some products. The peak blood levels of analgesics are achieved 30 minutes after taking a soluble dosage form; after a traditional *aspirin* tablet it may take up to 2 hours for peak levels to be reached.

The timing of doses may be important. With a migraine, the analgesic should be taken at the first sign of an attack, since GI motility is slowed during an attack and absorption of analgesics delayed. Combination therapy may sometimes be useful, for example an analgesic and decongestant (systemic or topical) in sinusitis.

The placebo effect is of great importance in pain relief, since the perception of pain is extremely subjective.

Aspirin

Aspirin is analgesic, antipyretic and also anti-inflammatory if given at doses greater than 4g daily. It should not be given to children under 12 years old because of its suspected link with Reye's syndrome. Recent reports indicate that some parents are still unaware of the contra-indication in children under 12 years old and deaths still occur from Reye's syndrome in young children as a result. Analgesics are often purchased for family use and it is worth reminding parents of the minimum age for *aspirin*'s use. It has been suggested that in addition to its use in the symptomatic treatment of headaches, doses of *aspirin* on alternate days may be effective in the prophylaxis of migraine.

Indigestion
Gastric irritation (indigestion, heartburn, nausea, vomiting) is sometimes experienced by patients after taking *aspirin* and for this reason the drug is best taken with or after food. When taken as soluble tablets, *aspirin* is less likely to cause gastric irritation and it is also available as an enteric-coated version which is designed so that the *aspirin* is released lower down the GI tract to try and prevent adverse effects. The pharmacist should remember though that enteric-coated preparations will not be released quickly and so they are inappropriate where rapid pain relief is required. The local use of *aspirin,* for example dissolving a soluble tablet near an aching tooth, is best avoided, since ulceration of the gums may result.

Bleeding
Aspirin can cause GI bleeding and should not be recommended for any patient who either currently has, or has a history of peptic ulcer. *Aspirin* effects the platelets and clotting function so that bleeding time is increased and it has been suggested that it should not be recommended for pain after tooth extraction for this reason. The effects of anticoagulant drugs are potentiated by *aspirin,* so it should never be recommended for patients taking these drugs.

Alcohol
Alcohol increases the irritant effect of *aspirin* on the stomach and also increases *aspirin*'s effects on bleeding time. Concurrent administration is therefore best avoided.

Pregnancy
Aspirin is best avoided in pregnancy.

Hypersensitivity
Hypersensitivity to *aspirin* occurs in some people; it has been estimated that 4% of asthmatic patients have this problem and *aspirin* should be avoided in any patient with a history of asthma. When such patients take *aspirin,* they may experience skin reactions (rashes, urticaria), or sometimes shortness of breath, bronchospasm and even asthma attacks.

Paracetamol
Paracetamol has analgesic and antipyretic effects but little or no anti-

inflammatory action. The exact way in which *paracetamol* exerts its analgesic effect remains unclear, despite extensive research. However, the drug is undoubtedly effective in reducing both pain and fever. *Paracetamol* is now the analgesic of choice for children under 12 years old and can be given to children from the age of 3 months onwards. It is less irritant to the stomach than *aspirin* and can therefore be recommended for those patients who are unable to take *aspirin* for this reason. A range of paediatric formulations, including sugar-free syrups, is available.

Liver toxicity

At high doses *paracetamol* can cause liver toxicity. This can be a problem after an overdose with *paracetamol,* since damage may not be apparent until a few days later. All overdoses of *paracetamol* should be taken seriously and the patient referred to a hospital casualty department.

Ibuprofen

Ibuprofen was transferred from the prescription only medicines (POM) list in 1984 and became available for sale OTC. It has analgesic, anti-inflammatory and antipyretic activity and causes less irritation and damage to the stomach than *aspirin*. The dose required for analgesic activity is 200–400 mg, that for anti-inflammatory action 300–600 mg. The maximum daily dose allowable for OTC use is 1200 mg and *ibuprofen* should not be given to children under 12 years old. *Ibuprofen* suspension 100 mg in 5 ml is available OTC. The doses are given 3 or 4 times daily and are: 1–2 years, 2.5 ml; 3–7 years, 5 ml; 8–12 years, 10 ml. The suspension is not to be given to children aged under 1 year old or weighing less than 16 lb, and should not be given to children who have asthma without checking with the doctor. As in adults, *ibuprofen* should not be given to children with a stomach ulcer or other serious stomach problem.

Indigestion

Ibuprofen can be irritant to the stomach, causing indigestion, nausea and diarrhoea, but less so than *aspirin*. Gastric bleeding can also occur. For these reasons, it is best to advise patients to take *ibuprofen* with or after food and it is best avoided in anyone with a peptic ulcer or a history of peptic ulcer. Elderly patients seem to be particularly prone to these effects and pharmacists should exercise care if recommending *ibuprofen* for such patients. *Ibuprofen* can increase the bleeding time due to an effect on platelets. This effect is reversible within 24 hours of stopping the drug (whereas reversibility may take several days after stopping *aspirin*).

Ibuprofen seems to have little or no effect on whole blood clotting or prothrombin time, but is still not advised for patients taking anticoagulant medication for whom *paracetamol* would be a better choice.

Hypersensitivity

Cross-sensitivity between *aspirin* and *ibuprofen* occurs, so it would be wise for the pharmacist not to recommend its use for anyone with a previous sensitivity reaction to *aspirin*. Since asthmatic patients are more likely to have such a reaction, the use of *ibuprofen* in asthmatic patients should be with caution.

Contra-indications

Sodium and water retention may be caused by *ibuprofen* and it is therefore best avoided in patients with congestive heart failure or renal impairment.

Ibuprofen is best avoided during pregnancy, particularly during the third trimester. Breastfeeding mothers may safely take *ibuprofen*, since it is excreted in only tiny amounts in the breastmilk.

Interactions

There is evidence of an interaction between *ibuprofen* and *lithium*. *Ibuprofen* may inhibit prostaglandin synthesis in the kidneys and reduce *lithium* clearance. Serum levels of *lithium* are thus raised, with the possibility of toxic effects. *Lithium* toxicity manifests itself as GI symptoms, polyuria, muscle weakness, lethargy and tremor.

Caution

Ibuprofen is best avoided in *aspirin*-sensitive patients and should be used with caution in asthmatics. Adverse effects are more likely to occur in the elderly and *paracetamol* may be a better choice in these cases.

Codeine

Codeine is a narcotic analgesic; a dose of at least 15 mg is required for analgesic effect. *Codeine* is commonly found in combination products with *aspirin, paracetamol* or both. Constipation is a possible side effect and is more likely in elderly patients and others prone to constipation. *Codeine* can also cause drowsiness and respiratory depression although this may be unlikely at OTC doses.

Dihydrocodeine

Dihydrocodeine is related to *codeine* and has similar analgesic efficacy. A combination product containing *paracetamol* and *dihydrocodeine* became available in the UK in 1992, with a dose per tablet of 7.46 mg *dihydrocodeine.* The product is restricted to use in adults and children over 12 years old. Side effects include constipation and drowsiness. Like *codeine,* the drug may cause respiratory depression at high doses.

Caffeine

Caffeine is included in some combination analgesic products to produce wakefulness and increased mental activity. It is probable that doses of at least 100 mg are needed to produce such an effect and that a cup of tea or coffee would have the same action. Products containing *caffeine* are best avoided near bedtime because of their stimulant effect. It has been claimed that *caffeine* increases the effectiveness of analgesics but the evidence for such claims is not definitive. *Caffeine* has an irritant effect on the stomach.

Doxylamine succinate

Doxylamine is an antihistamine whose sedative and relaxing effects are probably responsible for its usefulness in treating tension headaches. Like other older antihistamines, *doxylamine* can cause drowsiness and patients should be warned about this. *Doxylamine* should not be recommended for children under 12 years of age.

Buclizine and cyclizine

Buclizine and *cyclizine* are antihistamines which are used in OTC compound analgesics for their anti-emetic action. For this reason, they are included in some combination preparations for the treatment of migraine where nausea and vomiting is a problem. *Cyclizine* is well known as a drug of abuse. Pharmacists need to be aware that some drug misusers will seek to purchase it, even in compound products.

Feverfew

Feverfew is a herb which has been used in the prophylaxis of migraine. Some clinical trials have been conducted to examine its effectiveness, but results have been conflicting. However, the herb appears to be a promising agent in preventing migraines and also perhaps in diminishing the severity of symptoms when a migraine does occur. Adverse effects which have been reported from the use of feverfew include mouth ulceration involving the oral mucosa and tongue (which seems to occur in some 10% of patients), abdominal colic, heartburn and skin rashes. These effects occur both with feverfew leaves and when the herb is formulated in capsules. The herb has a bitter taste which some patients cannot tolerate. Feverfew was used in the past as an abortifacient and it should not be recommended for pregnant women with migraine.

Headaches in practice

Case 1

For several years Sandra Brown, a young mother, has purchased combination analgesics for migraine from your pharmacy every few months. She has suffered from migraine headaches since she was a child. Today she asks if you have anything stronger; the tablets do not seem to work like they used to. She is not taking any medicines on prescription (you check whether she is taking the contraceptive pill and she is not). Sandra tells you that she now suffers from migraines two or three times a month and they are making her life a misery. Nothing seems to trigger them and the pain is not more severe than before. She has read about feverfew and wonders whether she should give it a try.

The pharmacist's view

This woman has successfully used an OTC product to treat her migraines for a long period of time. Many patients who suffer migraines report that they get relief from OTC analgesics. Sandra's migraines have become more frequent for no apparent reason. Feverfew can be effective in preventing migraine in some patients. It would, however, be sensible to refer her to the doctor to exclude any serious cause of her headaches before considering further treatments.

The doctor's view

Prophylactic treatments (*propranolol* and *pizotifen*) for migraine are available and are worth considering in patients who report attacks more than once or twice a month. *Sumatriptan*, *zolmitriptan* and *naratriptan* are effective acute treatments for migraine, producing relief from a headache within an hour or two for many patients.

Case 2

A woman aged about 30 has asked to speak to you. She tells you that she would like you to recommend something for the headaches which she has been getting recently. You ask her to describe the headache and she explains that the pain is across her forehead and around the back of the head. The headaches usually occur during the daytime and have been occurring several times a week, for several weeks. There are no associated GI symptoms and there is no nasal congestion. No medicines are being taken, apart from a compound OTC product containing *aspirin*, which she has been taking for her headaches. On questioning her about recent changes in lifestyle, she tells you that she has recently moved to the area and started a new job last month. In the past she has suffered from the occasional headache, but not regularly. This lady does not wear glasses and says she has not had trouble with her eyesight in the past. She confides that she has been worried that the headaches might be due to something serious.

The pharmacist's view

From the information obtained, it sounds as though this woman is suffering from tension headaches. The location of the pain and lack of associated symptoms lead towards this conclusion. The timing of the headaches indicates that this woman's recent move and change of employment are probably responsible for the problem. The pharmacist should obtain information about the current headaches in relation to the patient's past experience. This patient is worried that the headaches may signal a serious problem, but the evidence indicates this would be unlikely. The pharmacist could recommend the use of a *paracetamol/ doxylamine* combination, warning about the possibility of drowsiness being induced by the antihistamine. If the headaches do not improve within a week she should see her doctor.

The doctor's view

The pharmacist's assessment is very reasonable. A tension headache is the most likely explanation. Hopefully, the reassurance and suggested treatment would help her symptoms within the week.

Case 3

Linda Vale is a regular visitor to your shop. She is a young mother, aged about 25 and today she seeks your advice about headaches which have been troubling her recently. The headaches are of a migraine type, quite severe and affecting one side of the head. Mrs Vale had her second child a few months ago and when you ask if she is taking any medicines she tells you that she recently started to take the combined oral contraceptive pill. In the past she has suffered from migraine-type headaches, but only occasionally and never as severe as the ones she has been experiencing during the past weeks. The headaches have been occurring once or twice a week for about 2 weeks. *Paracetamol* has given some relief, but Mrs Vale would like to try something stronger.

The pharmacist's view

Mrs Vale should be referred to her doctor immediately. Her history of migraine headaches associated with the oral contraceptive pill is a cause for concern, in addition you have established that she has suffered from migraine headaches in the past.

The doctor's view

The pharmacist should recommend referral to the doctor. Someone who develops their first migraine attack whilst taking the pill should be told to discontinue taking it. If there is a previous history of migraine the pill may sometimes be used, but if the frequency or severity of the migraines worsens on the pill, then once again the pill should be discontinued. The reason for this advice is that the migraine could herald a cerebral thrombosis (stroke) which could be prevented by stopping the pill. This advice should be given with both the progesterone-only and combined pills.

Musculoskeletal problems

Pharmacists are frequently asked for advice about muscular injuries, sprains and strains. Simple practical advice combined with topical or systemic over-the-counter (OTC) treatment can be valuable. Sometimes patients who are already taking prescribed medicines for musculoskeletal problems will ask for advice. Here a careful assessment of compliance with prescribed medicines and the need for referral is important.

What you need to know
Age
Child, adult, elderly
Symptoms
Pain, swelling, site, duration
History
Injury
Medical conditions
Medication

Significance of questions and answers

Age

Age will influence the pharmacist's choice of treatment, but other reasons make consideration of the patient's age important. In elderly patients, a fall is more likely to result in a fracture; elderly women are particularly at risk because of osteoporosis. Referral to the local casualty department for X-rays may be the best course of action in such cases.

Symptoms and history

Injuries commonly occur as a result of a fall or other trauma and during physical activity such as lifting heavy loads or taking part in sport. Exact details of how the injury occurred should be established by the pharmacist.

Sprains and strains

Sprains. A sprain injury involves the overstretching of ligaments and/ or the joint capsule, sometimes with tearing. The most common sprain involves the lateral ankle ligament. Referral is the best course of action, so that the family practitioner or casualty department doctor can examine the affected area and consider whether a complete tearing of ligaments has occurred, particularly for knee injuries. With a partial tear the knee is often swollen and the patient experiences severe pain on movement. A complete tear may involve the tearing of the capsule itself. If this occurs, any blood or fluid can leak out into the surrounding tissues, so the knee may not appear swollen.

Strains. These are injuries where the muscle fibres are damaged by over-stretching and tearing. Sometimes the fibres within the muscle sheath are torn, sometimes the muscle sheath itself ruptures and bleeding occurs. Strains are most common in muscles that work over two joints, for example the hamstring. When the strain heals, fibrosis can occur, and the muscle becomes shortened. The muscle is then vulnerable to further damage.

Early mobilization, strengthening exercises and coordination exercises are all important after both sprains and strains. The return to full activity must occur gradually.

Muscle pain

Stiff and painful muscles may occur simply as a result of strenuous and unaccustomed work such as gardening, decorating or exercise and the resulting discomfort can be reduced by treatment with OTC medicines.

Bruising

Bruising as a result of injury is common and some products which minimize bruising are available OTC. The presence of bruising without apparent injury, or a description by the patient of a history of bruising more easily than usual, should alert the pharmacist to the possibility of a more serious condition. Spontaneous bruising may be symptomatic of an underlying blood disorder, resulting from an adverse drug reaction or other cause.

Head injury

Pain occurring as a result of head injury should always be viewed with suspicion and such patients are best referred for further investigation, particularly children.

Bursitis

Other musculoskeletal problems about which the pharmacist's advice might be sought include bursitis, which is inflammation of bursae. (This is the name given to tissues around joints and where bones move over one another. The function of bursae is to reduce friction during movement.) Examples of bursitis are 'housemaid's knee' and 'student's elbow'.

Fibrositis

Fibrositis (fibromyalgia) refers to muscular pain which may involve the lower back, base of the neck, shoulders, elbows and knees. This condition is thought to have a psychogenic component and may be aggravated by stress.

Frozen shoulder

Frozen shoulder is a common condition where the shoulder is stiff and painful. It is more prevalent in older patients. The shoulder pain sometimes radiates to the arm and is often worse at night. Patients can sometimes, but not always, relate the problem to injury, exertion or exposure to cold, but frozen shoulder may occur without apparent cause. The pain and limitation of movement are usually so severe that referral to the doctor is advisable.

Painful joints

Pain arising in joints (arthralgia) may be due to arthritis, for which there are many causes. The pain may be associated with swelling, overlying inflammation, stiffness, limitation of movement and deformity of the joint. A common cause of arthritis is osteoarthritis which is due to wear and tear of the joint. This often affects the knees and hips, especially in the older population. Another form of arthritis is rheumatoid arthritis, which is a more generalized illness caused by the body turning its defences upon itself. Other forms of arthritis can be caused by gout or infection. A joint infection is rare but devastating and occasionally fatal. It is often difficult to distinguish between the different causes and it is therefore necessary to refer to the doctor except in mild cases.

Back pain

Lower back pain probably affects most people at some stage in their lives, often recurrently. Lower back pain which is not too severe or debilitating and comes on after gardening, awkward lifting or bending may be due to muscular strain (lumbago) and appropriate advice may be given by the pharmacist. If there is no improvement within a week following such advice, then referral is advisable.

Pain that is more severe, causing difficulty with mobility or radiating from the back down one or both legs, is an indication for referral. A slipped disc can press upon the sciatic nerve (hence 'sciatica') causing pain and sometimes 'pins and needles' and numbness in the leg.

Back pain which is felt in the middle to upper part of the back is less common and if it has been present for several days it is best referred to the doctor. Kidney pain can be felt in the back, to either side of the middle part of the back just below the ribcage. If the back pain is associated with any abnormality of passing urine (discoloration of urine, pain on passing urine, or frequency) then a kidney problem is more likely.

Repetitive strain disorder

This term covers several arm conditions, mainly affecting the forearm. 'Tenosynovitis' is the term which has been used to refer to conditions around the wrist which sometimes occur in Visual Display Unit (VDU) operators. The condition presents as swelling on the back of the forearm. There may be crepitus (a creaking, grating sound) when the wrist is moved. Sometimes the symptoms disappear on stopping the job, but they may return when the work is started again.

Whiplash injuries

Neck pain following a car accident can last for a long period; up to 2 years in some cases. Good posture is important and keeping both the back and head straight has been shown to reduce pain and help recovery. A physiotherapist's advice would probably include the recommendation to sleep with only one pillow to facilitate extension of the neck.

Medication

Prescribed medication

Sufferers of, for example, rheumatoid arthritis or chronic back pain are likely to be taking painkillers or non-steroidal anti-inflammatory drugs (NSAIDs) prescribed by their doctor. Although the recommendation of a topical analgesic would produce no problems in terms of drug interactions, if the patient is in considerable and regular pain despite prescribed medication, or the pain has become worse, referral back to the doctor would be appropriate.

Side effects. In the context of elderly patients, it should be remembered that falls may occur as a result of postural hypotension, dizziness or confusion as adverse effects from drug therapy. Any elderly patient reporting falls should be carefully questioned about current medication and the pharmacist should contact the doctor should an adverse reaction be suspected.

Self-medication

The pharmacist should also enquire about any preparations used in self-treatment of the condition and their degree of effectiveness.

Treatment timescale

Musculoskeletal conditions should respond to treatment within a few days. A maximum of 5 days' treatment should be recommended, after which patients should see their doctor.

Management

A wide range of preparations containing systemic and topical analgesics is available (see p. 183 for discussion of systemic analgesics). The oral analgesic of choice would usually be an NSAID such as *ibuprofen*, providing there were no contra-indications. Topical formulations include creams, ointments, lotions, sticks and sprays.

Topical analgesics

There is a high placebo response to topical analgesic products. This is probably because the act of massaging the formulation into the affected area will increase blood flow and stimulate the nerves, leading to a reduction in the sensation of pain.

Counter-irritants and rubefacients

Counter-irritants and rubefacients cause vasodilation, inducing a feeling of warmth over the area of application. Counter-irritants produce mild skin irritation and the term 'rubefacient' refers to the reddening and warming of the skin. The theory behind the use of topical analgesics is that they bombard the nervous system with sensations other than pain (warmth, irritation) and this is thought to 'distract attention' from the pain felt. Simply rubbing or massaging the affected area produces sensations of warmth and pressure and can reduce pain. Massage is known to relax muscles and it has also been suggested that massage may disperse some of the chemicals which are responsible for producing pain and inflammation by increasing the blood flow. The mode of action of topical analgesics is therefore twofold, one effect relying on absorption of the agent through the skin, the other on the effect of the massage.

There are many proprietary formulations available, often incorporating a mixture of ingredients with different properties. Most pharmacists and customers have their own favourite product. For customers who live alone, a spray formulation which does not require massage can be recommended for areas such as the back and shoulders.

Generally, patients can be advised to use topical analgesic products up to four times a day, as required.

Methyl salicylate

Methyl salicylate is one of the most widely used and effective counter-irritants. Wintergreen is the naturally occurring form of *methyl salicylate*; synthetic versions are also available. The agent is generally used in concentrations of between 10 and 60% in topical analgesic formulations.

Nicotinates

Nicotinates (e.g. *ethyl nicotinate, hexyl nicotinate*) are absorbed through the skin and produce reddening of the skin, increased blood flow and an increase in temperature. *Methyl nicotinate* is used at concentrations of 0.25–1% to produce its counter-irritant and rubefacient effects. There have been occasional reports of systemic adverse effects following absorption of nicotinates. Such effects may include dizziness or feelings of faintness and are due to a drop in blood pressure following vasodilation. However, systemic adverse effects are rare, they seem to occur only in susceptible people and are usually due to use of the product over a large surface area.

Menthol

Menthol has a cooling effect when applied to the skin and acts as a mild counter-irritant. Used in topical formulations in concentrations of up to 1%, *menthol* has antipruritic actions, but at higher concentrations it has a counter-irritant effect. When applied to the skin in a topical analgesic formulation, *menthol* gives a feeling of cooling, followed by a sensation of warmth.

Camphor

In concentrations up to 3%, *camphor* has antipruritic actions, in higher concentrations it acts as a counter-irritant and rubefacient. *Camphor* is highly toxic if swallowed and problems of toxicity led to the withdrawal from sale of some well-known formulations including *camphorated oil*.

Capsaicin/capsicum

The sensation of 'hotness' from eating peppers is caused by the excitation of nerve endings in the skin, body organs and airways. *Capsicum* preparations, for example *capsaicin capsicum* and *capsicum oloeoresin*, produce a feeling of warmth when applied to the skin. They do not cause reddening because they do not act on capillary or other blood vessels. *Capsaicin* has been the subject of recent research in clinical trials as an analgesic for post-herpetic pain and this work is continuing. Studies in patients with arthritis have also shown effectiveness. *Capsaicin* has few side effects. A small amount needs to be rubbed well into the affected area. Patients should always wash their hands afterwards, otherwise they may inadvertently transfer the substance to the eyes, causing burning and stinging.

Turpentine oil

Turpentine oil has counter-irritant and rubefacient actions and is a traditional ingredient of many topical analgesic formulations. It is the main ingredient of *white liniment BP*. It is used in concentrations of between 6 and 50%.

Topical anti-inflammatory agents

Topical gels, creams and ointments containing NSAIDs are widely used in the UK. Clinical trials have shown them to be more effective than placebo in relieving musculoskeletal pain. However there have been no comparative trials with counter-irritants and rubefacients.

Ibuprofen, felbinac, ketoprofen and *piroxicam* are available in a range of cream and gel formulations. The drug is absorbed into the bloodstream and appears to become concentrated in the affected tissues. Topical NSAIDs (except *benzydamine*) should not be used by patients who experience adverse reactions to *aspirin* such as asthma, rhinitis or urticaria. Because of the higher likelihood of *aspirin* sensitivity in patients with asthma, caution should be exercised when considering recommending a topical NSAID. Several reports of bronchospasm have been received following the use of these products. Rarely, gastrointestinal (GI) side effects have occurred, mainly dyspepsia, nausea and diarrhoea.

Heparinoid and hyaluronidase

These are enzymes which may help to disperse oedematous fluid in swollen areas. A reduction in swelling and bruising may therefore be achieved. Products containing *heparinoid* or *hyaluronidase* are used in the treatment of bruising, strains and sprains.

Practical points

First aid treatment of sprains and strains

As soon as possible after the injury has occurred, an ice-pack should be applied. Its function is to produce vasoconstriction, thus preventing further blood flow into the injured area from the torn capillaries and in turn minimizing further bruising and swelling. Proprietary cold-packs are available, but in emergencies various items have been brought into service. A bag of frozen peas, for example, is an excellent cold-pack for the knee or ankle because it can be easily applied and wrapped around the affected joint.

The affected limb should be elevated to reduce blood flow into the damaged area by the effect of gravity. This will, in turn, reduce the amount of swelling caused by oedema. The third piece of advice which the pharmacist can give is to apply compression to the injured area using a bandage. Finally, the injured limb should be rested to facilitate recovery. The acronym 'RICE' is a useful *aide-mémoire* for the treatment of sprains and strains.

R   Rest
I   Ice
C   Compression
E   Elevation

Heat

There is no doubt that the application of heat can be effective in reducing pain and is a simple method of pain relief. However, heat should never be applied immediately after an injury has occurred. This is because heat application at the acute stage will dilate blood vessels and increase blood flow into the affected area—the opposite effect to that which is needed.

After the acute phase is over (a day or two after the injury), heat can be useful. The application of heat can be both comforting and effective in chronic conditions such as back pain.

Patients can use a hot-water bottle, a proprietary heat-pack or an infrared lamp on the affected area. Heat-packs contain a mixture of chemicals which give off heat and the packs are disposable. Keeping the joints and muscles warm can also be helpful and the wearing of warm clothing, particularly in thin layers which can retain heat, is valuable.

Irritant effect of topical analgesics

Preparations containing topical analgesics should always be kept well away from the eyes, mouth and mucous membranes and should not be applied to broken skin. Intense pain and irritant effects can occur following such contact. This is due to the ready penetration of the irritant topical analgesics through both mucosal surfaces and direct access, via the broken skin. It should be remembered that when preparations are applied to thinner and more sensitive areas of the skin, irritant effects will be increased, hence the restrictions on the use of topical analgesics in young children recommended by some manufacturers for their products. Therefore, the manufacturer's instructions and recommendations should be checked.

Sensitization to counter-irritants can occur; if blistering or intense irritation of the skin results after application, the patient should discontinue use of the product.

Musculoskeletal problems in practice

Case 1

A middle-aged man comes into your shop. He is wearing a tracksuit and training shoes and asks what you can recommend for an aching back. On questioning, you find out that the product is in fact required for his wife, who was doing some gardening yesterday because the weather was fine and who now feels stiff and aching. The pain is in the lower back and is worse on movement. His wife is not taking any medicines on a regular basis but took two *paracetamol* last night, which helped to reduce the pain.

The pharmacist's view

In this case it would have been very easy for the pharmacist to assume that the man in the shop was also the patient whereas, in fact, he was making a request on his wife's behalf. This emphasizes the importance of establishing the identity of the patient. The history which is described is that of a common problem; muscle stiffness following unaccustomed or strenuous activity, in this case gardening. The pharmacist might recommend a combination of systemic and topical therapy. If there was an adequate supply of *paracetamol* tablets at home, the woman could continue to take a maximum of two tablets four times daily until the pain resolved. Alternatively, an anti-inflammatory agent such as *ibuprofen* could be advised, after checking that there were no contra-indications to its use. In addition, a topical rub or spray containing counter-irritants would help to warm the area and reduce pain. The woman should see her doctor if the symptoms have not improved within 5 days.

The doctor's view

The story is suggestive of simple muscle strain which should settle with the pharmacist's advice within a few days. It would be helpful to inquire whether or not she has had backaches before and, if so, what happened. It would also be worth checking that she did not have pain or 'pins and needles' radiating down her legs. If these symptoms were present then she might have a slipped disc and referral to her doctor would be advisable.

Case 2

An elderly female customer who regularly visits your pharmacy asks what would be the best thing for rheumatic pain which is worse now that the weather is getting colder. The pain is in the joints, particularly of the fingers and knees. On further questioning, you find out that she has suffered from this problem for some years and that she sees her doctor quite regularly about this and a variety of other complaints. On checking your patient medication records you find that she is taking five different medicines a day. Her regular medication includes a combination diuretic preparation, sleeping tablets and analgesics for her arthritis (Co-Dydramol plus a NSAID). The joint pains seem to have become worse during the recent spell of bad weather.

The pharmacist's view

It would be best for this customer to see her doctor. She is already taking several medicines, including analgesics for arthritis. It would therefore be inappropriate for the pharmacist to consider recommendation of a systemic anti-inflammatory or analgesic because of the possibilities of interaction or duplication. Indeed, the recent worsening of the symptoms indicates that consultation with the doctor would be wise. Perhaps this woman is not taking all her medicines; the pharmacist could explore any compliance problems with her before referring her back to the doctor.

The doctor's view

Referral to the doctor is advisable. She may have osteoarthritis, rheumatoid arthritis or even some other form of arthritis and the doctor would be in the best position to advise further treatment.

Women's Health

Cystitis

Cystitis is common in women but rare in men; it has been estimated that more than one in two women will experience an episode of cystitis during their lives. The symptoms of cystitis may be due to a bacterial infection in about half the cases and the pharmacist should be aware of the signs which indicate more serious conditions. Over-the-counter (OTC) products are available for the treatment of cystitis, but are recommended only when symptoms are mild, or for use until patients can consult their doctor.

What you need to know

Age
    Adult, child
Male or female
Symptoms
    Urethral irritation
    Urinary urgency, frequency
    Dysuria (pain on passing urine)
    Haematuria (blood in the urine)
    Vaginal discharge
Associated symptoms
    Back pain
    Lower abdominal (suprapubic) pain
    Fever, chills
    Nausea/vomiting
Duration
Previous history
Medication

Significance of questions and answers

Age

Any child with the symptoms of cystitis should always be referred to the doctor for further investigation and treatment. Urinary tract infections (UTIs) occur in children and damage to the kidney or bladder may result, particularly after recurrent infections.

Gender

Cystitis is much more common in women than in men for two reasons.

First, cystitis occurs when bacteria pass up along the urethra and enter and multiply within the bladder. As the urethra is much shorter in females than in males, the passage of the bacteria is much easier. In addition the process is facilitated by sexual intercourse.

Second, there is evidence that prostatic fluid has antibacterial properties, providing an additional defence against bacterial infection in males.

Referral

Any man who presents with the symptoms of cystitis requires medical referral because of the possibility of more serious conditions such as kidney or bladder stones, or prostate problems.

Pregnancy

If a pregnant woman presents with symptoms of cystitis, referral to the doctor is the best option, because bacteruria (presence of bacteria in the urine) in pregnancy can lead to kidney infection and other problems.

Symptoms

Cystitis sufferers often report that the first sign of an impending attack is an itching or pricking sensation in the urethra. The desire to pass urine becomes frequent and women with cystitis may feel the need to pass urine urgently, but pass only a few burning, painful drops. This frequency of urine occurs throughout the day and night. Dysuria (pain on passing urine) is a classical symptom of cystitis. After urination, the bladder may not feel completely empty, but even straining produces no further flow.

The urine may be cloudy and strong-smelling; these may be signs of bacterial infection.

Blood in urine

The presence of blood in the urine (haematuria) is an indication for referral to the doctor. It often occurs in cystitis when there is so much inflammation of the lining of the bladder and urethra that bleeding occurs. This is not serious and responds quickly to antibiotic treatment. Sometimes blood in the urine may indicate other problems such as a kidney stone. When this occurs, pain in the loin or between the loin and groin is the predominant symptom. When blood in the urine develops without any pain then specialist referral is required to exclude the possibility of a tumour in the bladder or kidney.

Vaginal discharge

The presence of a vaginal discharge would indicate local fungal or bacterial infection and would require referral.

Associated symptoms

When dealing with symptoms involving the urinary system it is best to think of it as divided into two parts: the upper (kidneys and ureters); and the lower (bladder and urethra). The pharmacist should be aware of the symptoms which accompany minor lower UTI and those which suggest more serious problems higher in the urinary tract, so that referral for medical advice can be made where appropriate.

Upper urinary tract infection symptoms

Systemic involvement, demonstrated by fever, nausea, vomiting, loin pain and tenderness are indicative of more serious infection such as pyelitis or pyelonephritis and patients with such symptoms require referral.

Other symptoms

Cystitis may be accompanied by suprapubic (lower abdominal) pain and tenderness; pain is sometimes felt in the lower back.

Duration

Treatment with OTC preparations is reasonable for mild cystitis of short duration (less than 2 days).

Previous history

Women with recurrent cystitis should see their doctor, since repeated UTI can lead to kidney damage and even renal failure. One in two episodes of cystitis is not caused by infection and the 'urethral syndrome' is thought to be responsible for these non-infective cases. The anxiety produced by repeated occurrences of cystitis is thought to be a contributory factor itself.

It has been estimated that one in 10 cases of UTI is followed by relapse (the same bacterium being responsible) or reinfection (where a different organism may be involved). The remaining nine in 10 cases clear up without recurrence.

Diabetes

Recurrent cystitis can sometimes occur in diabetic patients and anyone describing a history of increasing thirst, weight loss and a higher frequency of passing urine than normal should be referred for this reason.

Honeymoon cystitis

Sexual intercourse may precipitate an attack ('honeymoon' cystitis) due to minor trauma or resulting infection when bacteria are pushed along the urethra.

Other precipitating factors

These are thought to include the irritant effects of toiletries (e.g. bubble baths and vaginal deodorants) and other chemicals (e.g. spermicides and disinfectants). Lack of personal hygiene is not thought to be responsible, except in extreme cases.

Postmenopausal women

Oestrogen deficiency in postmenopausal women leads to thinning of the lining of the vagina. Lack of lubrication can mean the vagina and urethra are vulnerable to trauma and irritation and attacks of cystitis can occur. For such women, painful intercourse can also be a problem and this can be treated with OTC lubricants or prescribed products (e.g. oestrogen creams). Lubricant products are available OTC and newer formulations mean that a single application can remain effective for several days. Should this approach not be successful, or if other troublesome symptoms are present, referral to the doctor would be advisable.

Medication

Cystitis can be caused by cytotoxic drugs such as *cyclophosphamide* and *hexamine* (because of formaldehyde release). It has been claimed that the incidence of cystitis is higher in women who are on the pill. However no causative effect has ever been shown. It has been suggested that since women taking the pill are more likely to be sexually active,this may explain the difference in incidence of cystitis.

The identity of any preparations already taken to treat the symptoms is therefore important. The pharmacist may then decide whether an appropriate remedy has been used. Failed medication would be a reason for referral to the doctor.

When to refer
All men, children
Fever, nausea/vomiting
Loin pain or tenderness
Haematuria
Vaginal discharge
Duration of longer than 2 days
Pregnancy
Recurrent cystitis
Failed medication

Treatment timescale

If symptoms have not subsided within 2 days of beginning treatment, the patient should see her doctor.

Management

In general, the pharmacist can recommend a product which will alkalinize the urine and provide symptomatic relief. Other OTC preparations are of doubtful value. In addition to treatment, it is important for the pharmacist to offer advice about fluid intake (see *Practical points* below). For women in whom cystitis is a recurrent problem, self-help measures can sometimes prevent recurrence. Literature can be offered on this subject.

Potassium and sodium citrate

These substances work by making the urine alkaline. The acidic urine produced as a result of bacterial infection is thought to be responsible for dysuria; alkalinization of the urine can therefore provide symptomatic relief. While easing discomfort, alkalinizing the urine will not produce an antibacterial effect and it is important to tell patients that if symptoms have not improved within 2 days, they should see their doctor.

Contra-indications

Formulary and proprietary preparations are available and can be effective in easing discomfort. However, there are some patients for whom such preparations should not be recommended. For *potassium citrate* these would include anyone taking potassium-sparing diuretics, aldosterone antagonists or angiotensin-converting enzyme (ACE) inhibitors, in whom hyperkalaemia may result. *Sodium citrate* should not be recommended for hypertensive patients, anyone with heart disease, or pregnant women.

Advice

Potassium citrate mixture tastes unpleasant, despite its fruity lemon smell and patients should be advised to dilute the mixture well with cold water.

Warning

Patients should be reminded not to exceed the stated dose of products containing *potassium citrate*: several cases of hyperkalaemia have been reported in patients taking *potassium citrate mixture* for relief from urinary symptoms.

Practical points

1 Drinking large quantities of fluids can help in cystitis because the bladder is emptied more frequently and completely as a result of the diuresis produced; this is thought to help flush the infecting bacteria out of the bladder. Soft drinks such as barley water are said to be of particular help.

2 The Health Education Authority (HEA) produces useful leaflets about cystitis. Copies can be obtained by pharmacists from the HEA itself, or via district health promotion units.

3 There are several paperbacks published on the subject of cystitis, including Angela Kilmartin's *Cystitis—A Self-help Guide* (Arrow Publications, London).

4 Reduced intake of coffee and alcohol may help because these substances seem to act as bladder irritants in some people.

5 Patients should be advised to routinely ensure that the bladder is fully emptied by waiting for 20 seconds after passing urine and then straining to empty the final drops. After a bowel motion the toilet paper should be wiped from front to back to minimize transfer of bacteria from the bowel into the vagina and urethra. Emptying of the bladder 15 minutes after sexual intercourse can help to prevent infection.

6 Cranberry juice has been recommended as a folk remedy for years as a preventive measure to reduce urinary tract infections. There is some evidence from a clinical trial in elderly women that drinking cranberry juice on a regular basis (300 ml per day) has a bacteriostatic effect. The mechanism for this is unknown and the full clinical implications have not been elucidated. For women who are prone to cystitis, drinking cranberry juice is not harmful and might help.

Cystitis in practice

Case 1

Mrs Anne Lawson, a young woman in her twenties, asks to have a quiet word with you. She tells you she thinks she has cystitis. Upon questioning, you find that she is not passing urine more frequently than normal, but that her urine looks dark and smells unpleasant. Mrs Lawson has back pain and has been feeling feverish during today. She is not taking any medicine from the doctor and has not tried anything to treat her symptoms.

The pharmacist's view

This woman has described symptoms which are not of a minor nature. In particular, the presence of fever and back pain indicates an infection higher in the urinary tract. Mrs Lawson should see her doctor as soon as possible.

The doctor's view

Referral is advisable. She may have a UTI, possibly in the kidney. However, there is insufficient information to make a definite diagnosis. It would be useful to know if she has pain on passing urine and the site and nature of her back pain. Her symptoms could in fact be accounted for by a flu-like viral infection in which the backache is caused by muscular inflammation and the urine altered because of dehydration.

Case 2

A young man asks if you can recommend a good treatment for cystitis. In response to your questions, he tells you that the medicine is for him: he has been having pain when passing urine since yesterday. He feels otherwise well and does not have any other symptoms. No treatments have been tried already and he is not currently taking any medicines.

The pharmacist's view

This man should be referred to the doctor because the symptoms of cystitis are uncommon in men and may be the result of a more serious condition.

The doctor's view

Referral is necessary for accurate diagnosis. A urine sample will need to be collected for appropriate analysis. If it shows that he has a urinary infection then treatment with a suitable antibiotic can be given and a referral to a specialist for further investigation made. If in addition to discomfort on passing urine he develops a urethral discharge, he is most likely to be suffering from a sexually transmitted disease such as non-specific urethritis (NSU) or gonorrhoea.

Case 3

It is Saturday afternoon and a young woman whom you do not recognize as a regular customer asks for something to treat cystitis. On questioning, you find out that she has had the problem several times before and that her symptoms are frequency and pain on passing urine. She is otherwise well and tells you that her doctor has occasionally prescribed antibiotics to treat the problem in the past. She is not taking any medicines.

The pharmacist's view

This woman represents a common situation in community pharmacy. She has had these symptoms before and is unlikely to be able to see her doctor before Monday. In the meantime she is experiencing considerable discomfort. It would be reasonable to recommend the use of an alkalinizing agent, such as *sodium* or *potassium citrate*, over the weekend. Proprietary formulations are more pleasant tasting than the *potassium citrate mixture* and they are very acceptable to patients. You could advise her to drink plenty of fluids but with minimum consumption of tea, coffee and alcohol, all of which may cause dehydration and make the problem worse. An emergency supply of the antibiotic which has been prescribed for her in the past might be a possibility, providing the antibiotic could be identified and that the legal requirements for emergency supplies were met. She should see her doctor on Monday if the symptoms have not improved.

The doctor's view

The story is suggestive of cystitis. Symptomatic treatment with *potassium citrate* may help until after the weekend. It would be interesting to know how her infections usually resolve. If she had severe symptoms it would be reasonable to start treatment with an antibiotic. If there was any doubt as to the type of treatment, many on-call doctors are willing to give advice over the phone.

Dysmenorrhoea

It has been estimated that as many as one in two women suffer from dysmenorrhoea (period pains). Up to one in 10 of those affected will have severe symptoms which necessitate time off school or work. Many of these women will try self-medication, seeking advice from their doctor only if this treatment is unsuccessful. Pharmacists should remain aware that discussing menstrual problems is potentially embarrassing for the patient and should therefore try to create an atmosphere of privacy.

What you need to know

Age
Previous history
    Regularity and timing of cycle
Timing and nature of pains
    Relationship with menstruation
Other symptoms
    Headache, backache
    Nausea, vomiting ,constipation
    Faintness, dizziness, fatigue
    Premenstrual syndrome (PMS)
Medication

Significance of questions and answers

Age

The peak incidence of primary dysmenorrhoea occurs in women between the ages of 17 and 25. Primary dysmenorrhoea is defined as pain in the absence of pelvic disease, whereas secondary dysmenorrhoea refers to pain which may be due to underlying disease. Secondary dysmenorrhoea is most common in women aged over 30 and is rare in women aged under 25. Common causes of secondary dysmenorrhoea include endometriosis or pelvic inflammatory disease (PID). Primary dysmenorrhoea is uncommon after having children.

Previous history

Dysmenorrhoea is often not associated with the start of menstruation (the menarche). This is because during the early months (and sometimes years) of menstruation, ovulation does not occur. These anovulatory cycles are usually, but not always, pain free and therefore women sometimes describe period pain which begins after several months or years of pain-free menstruation.

The pharmacist should establish whether the menstrual cycle is regular and the length of the cycle. Further questioning should then focus on the timing of pains in relation to menstruation.

Timing and nature of pains

Primary dysmenorrhoea

This classically presents as a cramping lower abdominal pain which often begins during the day before bleeding starts. The pain gradually eases after the start of menstruation and is often gone by the end of the first day of bleeding.

Mittelschmerz. Is ovulation pain which occurs mid-cycle, at the time of ovulation. The abdominal pain usually lasts for a few hours, but can last for several days and may be accompanied by some bleeding.

Secondary dysmenorrhoea

The pain of secondary or acquired dysmenorrhoea may occur during other parts of the menstrual cycle and can be relieved or worsened by menstruation. Such pain is often described as a dull, aching pain rather than being spasmodic or cramping in nature. Often occurring up to a week before menstruation, the pain may get worse once bleeding starts. The pain may occur during sexual intercourse. Secondary dysmenorrhoea is more common in older women, especially in those who have had children. In pelvic infection, a vaginal discharge may be present in addition to pain. If, from questioning, the pharmacist suspects secondary dysmenorrhoea, the patient should be referred to her doctor for further investigation.

Endometriosis. Endometriosis mainly occurs in women aged between 30 and 45, but can occur in women in their twenties. The womb (uterus) has a unique inner lining surface (endometrium). In endometriosis, pieces of endometrium are also found in places outside the uterus. These isolated pieces of endometrium may lie on the outside of the uterus or ovaries, or elsewhere in the pelvis. Each section of endometrium is sensitive to hormonal changes occurring during the menstrual cycle and goes through the monthly changes of thickening, shedding and bleeding. This causes pain wherever the endometrial cells are found. The pain usually begins up to a week before menstruation and both lower abdominal and lower back pain may occur. Mittelschmerz can be severe and the cycle can sometimes be shortened so that ovulation pain may be closely followed by premenstrual and menstrual pain. Once the flow of blood is established, pain may be relieved.

Pelvic inflammatory disease (PID). Pelvic infection can occur and may be acute or chronic in nature. It is important to know whether or not an intra-uterine contraceptive device (coil) is used. The coil can cause increased discomfort and heavier periods, but also may predispose to infection. Acute pelvic infection occurs when a bacterial infection develops within the Fallopian tubes. There is usually severe pain, fever and vaginal discharge. The pain is lower abdominal in situation and may be unrelated to menstruation. It may be confused with appendicitis.

Chronic PID may follow on from an acute infection. The pain tends to be less severe, associated with periods and may be experienced during intercourse. It is thought that adhesions which develop around the tubes following an infection may be responsible for the symptoms in some women. In others, however, no abnormality can be found and pelvic congestion is assumed to be the cause. In this situation psychological factors are thought to be important.

Other symptoms

Women who experience dysmenorrhoea will often describe other, associated symptoms. These include nausea, vomiting, general gastrointestinal (GI) discomfort, constipation, headache, backache, fatigue, feeling faint and dizziness.

Premenstrual syndrome (PMS)

The term 'premenstrual syndrome' describes a collection of symptoms, both physical and mental, whose incidence is related to the menstrual cycle. Symptoms are experienced cyclically, usually from 2 to 14 days before the start of menstruation. Relief from symptoms generally occurs once menstrual bleeding begins. The cyclical nature, timing and reduction in symptoms are all important in identifying PMS. Some women experience such severe symptoms that their working and home lives are affected.

Sufferers often complain of a bloated abdomen, increase in weight, swelling of ankles and fingers, breast tenderness and headaches. Women who experience PMS describe a variety of mental symptoms which may include any, or all of irritability, tension, depression, difficulty in concentrating and tiredness.

If PMS is considered to be a possibility, advising the woman to keep a diary of symptoms, recording when they occur and remit is useful, especially if the pharmacist later decides referral is needed.

Treatment of the symptoms of PMS is a matter for debate and there is a high placebo response to therapy of mood changes, breast discomfort and headaches when taken from 2 weeks before the period starts or throughout the cycle. There is some evidence that *pyridoxine* may reduce symptoms. The mechanism of action of *pyridoxine* in PMS is unknown. However, women should be advised to stick to the recommended dose; higher doses of *pyridoxine* are reported to have led to neuritis.

Evening primrose oil has been shown to be effective in reducing breast tenderness associated with PMS and may also reduce other symptoms. The mechanism of action of *evening primrose oil* in such cases is thought to be linked to effects on prostaglandins, particularly in increasing the level of prostaglandin E, which appears to be depleted in some women with PMS. The active component of *evening primrose oil* is gammalinolenic acid, which is thought to reduce the ratio of saturated to unsaturated fatty acids. The response to hormones and prolactin appears to be reduced by gammalinolenic acid.

Medication

The pain of dysmenorrhoea is thought to be linked to increased prostaglandin activity and raised prostaglandin levels have been found in the menstrual fluids and circulating blood of women who suffer from dysmenorrhoea. Therefore, the use of analgesics which inhibit the synthesis of prostaglandins is logical. It is important, however, for the pharmacist to make sure that the patient is not already taking a non-steroidal anti-inflammatory drug (NSAID).

Women taking oral contraceptives usually find that the symptoms of dysmenorrhoea are reduced or eliminated altogether and so any woman presenting with the symptoms of dysmenorrhoea and who is taking the pill is probably best referred to the doctor for further investigation.

When to refer
Presence of abnormal vaginal discharge
Abnormal bleeding
Symptoms suggest secondary dysmenorrhoea
Severe intermenstrual pain (mittelschmerz) and bleeding
Failure of medication
Pain with a late period (possibility of an early pregnancy)
Presence of fever

Treatment timescale

If the pain of primary dysmenorrhoea is not improved after two cycles' treatment, referral to the doctor would be advisable.

Management

Simple explanation about why period pains occur, together with sympathy and reassurance, is important. Treatment with simple analgesics is often very effective in dysmenorrhoea.

Ibuprofen (see also p. 185)

Ibuprofen can be considered the treatment of choice for dysmenorrhoea, providing the drug is appropriate for the patient (i.e. the pharmacist has questioned the patient about previous use of *aspirin,* and history of GI problems and asthma). *Ibuprofen* inhibits the synthesis of prostaglandins and thus has a rationale for use. For self-medication, a maximum daily dose of 1200 mg per day is allowed, so women could be advised to try a dose of 200–400 mg three times daily. A variety of proprietary brands of *ibuprofen* is available, in tablet and capsule form, some of which are specifically marketed for period pains. Sustained release formulations of *ibuprofen* are also available.

Contra-indications

Care should be taken when recommending *ibuprofen.* The drug can cause GI irritation and should not be taken by anyone who has or has had a peptic ulcer. All patients should take *ibuprofen* with or after food to minimize GI problems (also see p. 185).

Ibuprofen should not be taken by anyone who is sensitive to *aspirin* and should be used with caution in anyone who is asthmatic, because such patients are more likely to be sensitive to *ibuprofen.*

Aspirin

Aspirin also inhibits the synthesis of prostaglandins but is less effective in relieving the symptoms of dysmenorrhoea than *ibuprofen. Aspirin* can cause GI upsets and is more irritant to the stomach than *ibuprofen.* For those women who experience symptoms of nausea and vomiting with dysmenorrhoea, *aspirin* is probably best avoided for this reason. Soluble forms of *aspirin* will work more quickly than traditional tablet formulations and are less likely to cause stomach problems. Patients should be advised to take *aspirin* with or after meals.

The pharmacist should establish whether the patient has any history of *aspirin* sensitivity before recommending the drug.

Paracetamol

Paracetamol has little or no effect on the levels of prostaglandins involved in pain and inflammation and so it is theoretically less effective for the treatment of dysmenorrhoea than either *ibuprofen* or *aspirin*. However, *paracetamol* is a useful treatment when the patient cannot take *ibuprofen* or *aspirin* because of stomach problems or potential sensitivity. *Paracetamol* is also useful when the patient is suffering nausea and vomiting as well as pain, since it does not irritate the stomach. The pharmacist should remember to stress the maximum dose which can be taken.

Hyoscine/homatropine

These are smooth muscle relaxants which are included in some proprietary products marketed for the treatment of dysmenorrhoea on the theoretical basis that their antispasmodic action will reduce cramping. In fact, these drugs are included at such low doses (0.1 mg *hyoscine* in some combination formulations) that such an effect is unlikely and such products might be considered to be successful due to their analgesic action and their psychological effect. An over-the-counter (OTC) product containing 10 mg *hyoscine* is available. The anticholinergic effects of *hyoscine* mean it is contra-indicated in women with closed-angle glaucoma. Additive anticholinergic effects (dry mouth, constipation, blurred vision) means *hyoscine* is best avoided if any other drug with anticholinergic effects (e.g. tricyclic antidepressants) is being taken.

Caffeine

Caffeine is included in some proprietary products on the grounds that fatigue is often experienced by women with dysmenorrhoea. *Caffeine* undoubtedly has a stimulant effect, but a similar effect would be achieved through drinking tea or coffee. Patients who buy products containing *caffeine* should be reminded not to take them near bedtime, since these products may keep them awake.

Practical points

1 Exercise during menstruation is not harmful, as some 'old wives' tales' would have people believe. In fact, exercise may well be beneficial, since it raises endorphin levels, reducing pain and promoting a feeling of well-being.
2 Simple measures, like the use of a hot-water bottle, can help relieve abdominal and lower back pain.

Dysmenorrhoea in practice

Case 1

Linda Bailey is a young woman aged about 26, who asks your advice about painful periods. From your questioning, you find that Linda has lower abdominal pain and sometimes backache, which starts several days before her period begins. Her menstrual cycle used to be very regular, but now tends to vary; sometimes she only has 3 weeks between periods. The pain continues throughout menstruation and is quite severe. She has tried taking *aspirin*, which did not have much effect.

The pharmacist's view

This woman sounds as though she is experiencing secondary dysmenorrhoea—the pain begins well before her period starts and continues during menstruation. Her periods, which used to be regular, are no longer so and she has tried *aspirin* which has not relieved the pain. She should be referred to her doctor.

The doctor's view

Referral does seem appropriate in this situation. Further information needs to be gathered from history taking, examination and preliminary investigations. It is quite possible that the patient has endometriosis and referral to a gynaecologist may be indicated.

Case 2

Jenny Simmonds is a young woman aged about 18 who looks rather embarrassed and asks you what would be the best thing for period pains. Jenny tells you that she started her periods about 5 years ago and has never had any problem with period pains until recently. Her periods are regular; every 4 weeks. They have not become heavier, but she now gets pain which starts a few hours before her period. The pain has usually gone by the end of the first day of menstruation and Jenny has never had any pain during other parts of the cycle. She says she has not tried any medicine yet, is not taking any medicines from the doctor and that she can normally take *aspirin* without any problems.

The pharmacist's view

From the results of questioning, it sounds as though Jenny is suffering from straightforward primary dysmenorrhoea. She could be advised to take *ibuprofen*, 200–400 mg three times daily. She could be recommended to follow this regime for 2 months and invited back to see if the treatment has worked.

The doctor's view

Jenny's pain is most likely to be due to primary dysmenorrhoea. An explanation of this fact would probably be very reassuring. The treatment recommended by the pharmacist is sensible.

Vaginal thrush

Women often seek to buy products for 'feminine itching' and may be embarrassed to seek advice or answer what they see as intrusive questions from the pharmacist. Since 1992, vaginal pessaries and intravaginal creams containing *imidazole* antifungals have been available over the counter (OTC) from pharmacies in the UK. Oral *fluconazole* became available for OTC sale in 1995. The availability of these treatments offers the pharmacist an opportunity to provide effective therapy for vaginal thrush. Before making any recommendation it is vital to question the patient to identify the probable cause of the symptoms. Advertising of these treatments direct to the public means that a request for a named product may be made. It is important to confirm its appropriateness.

What you need to know

Age
   Child, adult, elderly
Duration
Symptoms
   Itch
   Soreness
   Discharge (colour, consistency, odour)
   Dysuria
   Dyspareunia
   Threadworms
Previous history
Medication

Significance of questions and answers

Age

Vaginal candidiasis (thrush) is common in women of child-bearing age and pregnancy and diabetes are strong predisposing factors. This infection is rare in children and in postmenopausal women because of the different environment in the vagina. In contrast to women of child-bearing age, where vaginal pH is generally acidic (low pH) and contains glycogen, the vaginal environment of children and menopausal women tends to be alkaline (high pH) and does not contain large amounts of glycogen.

Oestrogen, present between adolescence and the menopause, leads to the availability of glycogen in the vagina and also contributes to the development of a protective barrier layer on the walls of the vagina. The lack of oestrogen in children and postmenopausal women means this protective barrier is not present, with a consequent increased tendency to bacterial (but not fungal) infection.

In the UK, the Committee on Safety of Medicines recommends that women aged under 16 or over 60 complaining of symptoms of vaginal thrush should be referred to their doctor. Child abuse may be the source of vaginal infection in girls, making referral even more important. Vaginal thrush is rare in older women and other causes of the symptoms need to be excluded.

Duration

Some women delay seeking advice from the pharmacist or doctor because of embarrassment about their symptoms. They may have tried an OTC product or a prescription medicine already (see *Medication* below).

Symptoms

Itch (pruritus)

Dermatitis. Allergic or irritant dermatitis may be responsible for vaginal itch. It is worth asking about whether the patient has recently used any new toiletries (e.g. soaps, bath or shower products). Vaginal deodorants are sometimes the source of allergic reactions. Women sometimes use harsh soaps, antiseptics and vaginal douches in over-enthusiastic cleansing of the vagina. Regular washing with warm water is all that is required to keep the vagina clean and to maintain a healthy vaginal environment. *Candidiasis (thrush).* The itch associated with thrush is often intense and burning in nature. Sometimes the skin may be excoriated and raw from scratching when the itch is severe.

Discharge

In women of child-bearing age, the vagina naturally produces a watery discharge and cervical mucus is also produced, which changes consistency at particular times of the menstrual cycle. Such fluids may be watery or slightly thicker, with no associated odour. Some women worry about these natural secretions and think they have an infection.

The most common infective cause of vaginal discharge is candidiasis. Vaginal candidiasis may be (but is not always) associated with a discharge. The discharge is classically creamy-coloured, thick and curdy in appearance, but alternatively may be thin and rather watery. Other vaginal infections may be responsible for producing discharge but are markedly different from that caused by thrush. The discharge associated with candidal infection does not usually produce an unpleasant odour, in contrast to that produced by bacterial infection. Infection leading to discharge described as yellow or greenish is more likely to be bacterial in origin.

Partner's symptoms
Men may be infected with candida without showing any symptoms.

Dysuria (pain on urination)
Dysuria may be present and scratching the skin in response to itching might be responsible, although dysuria may occur without scratching. Sometimes, the pain on passing water may be mistaken for cystitis by the patient. If a woman complains of cystitis it is therefore important to ask about other symptoms (see p. 203). The UK Committee on Safety of Medicines advises that lower abdominal pain or dysuria are indications for referral because of their possible link with kidney infections.

Dyspareunia (painful intercourse)
Painful intercourse may be associated with infection or a sensitivity reaction where the vulval and vaginal areas are involved.

Threadworms
Occasionally, threadworm infestation can lead to vaginal pruritus and this has sometimes occurred in children. The patient would also be experiencing anal itching in such a case. The pharmacist should refer girls under the age of 16 to the doctor in any case of vaginal symptoms.

Previous history
Recurrent thrush is a problem for some women, often following antibiotic treatment (see below). Any woman who has experienced more than two attacks of thrush during the previous 6 months should be referred to the doctor. Repeated thrush infections may indicate an underlying problem or altered immunity and further investigation is needed.

Pregnancy
During pregnancy almost one in five women will have an episode of vaginal candidiasis. This high incidence has been attributed to hormonal changes with a consequent alteration in the vaginal environment leading to the presence of increased quantities of glycogen. Any pregnant woman with thrush should be referred to the doctor.

Diabetes

It is thought that candida is able to grow more easily in diabetic patients because of the higher glucose levels in blood and tissues. Sometimes recurrent vaginal thrush can be a sign of undiagnosed diabetes or, in a patient who has been diagnosed, of poor diabetic control.

Sexually transmitted diseases (STDs)

In the UK, the Committee on Safety of Medicines insists that women who have previously had a sexually transmitted infection should not be sold OTC treatments for thrush. The thinking behind this ruling is that with a previous history of STD, the current condition may not be thrush or may include a dual infection with another organism.

Pharmacists may be concerned about how patients will respond to 'personal' questions. However, it should be possible to enquire about previous episodes of these or similar symptoms in a tactful way, for example by asking 'Have you ever had anything like this before?' and if 'Yes', 'Tell me about the symptoms—were they exactly the same as this time?' and about the partner, 'Has your boyfriend/husband/partner mentioned any symptoms recently?'.

Oral steroids

Patients taking oral steroids may be at increased risk of candidal infection.

Immunocompromised patients

Patients with the human immunodeficiency virus (HIV) or acquired immune deficiency syndrome (AIDS) are prone to recurrent thrush infection because the immune system is unable to combat them. Patients undergoing cancer chemotherapy are also at risk of infection.

Medication

Oral contraceptives

Some experts have suggested that the oral contraceptive pill is linked to the incidence of vaginal candidiasis, however there is no convincing evidence that the link is due to physiological or pharmacological effects of the pill. The more likely reason for the apparent link is that women taking the pill are likely to be sexually active and not using a barrier method of contraception.

Antibiotics

Broad spectrum antibiotics wipe out the natural bacterial flora (lactobacilli) in the vagina and can predispose to candidal overgrowth. Some women find that an episode of thrush follows every course of antibiotics they take. The doctor may prescribe an antifungal at the same time as the antibiotic in such cases.

Local anaesthetics

Vaginal pruritus may actually be caused by some of the products used to relieve the symptom. Creams and ointments advertised for 'feminine' itching often contain local anaesthetics, a well-know cause of sensitivity reactions. It is important to check what, if any treatment the patient has tried before seeking your advice.

When to refer

The UK Committee on Safety of Medicines' list:
  First occurrence of symptoms
  Known hypersensitivity to imidazoles or other vaginal antifungal
    products
  Pregnancy or suspected pregnancy
  More than two attacks in the previous 6 months
  Previous history of STD
  Exposure to partner with STD
  Patient aged under 16 or over 60
  Abnormal or irregular vaginal bleeding
  Any blood staining of vaginal discharge
  Vulval or vaginal sores, ulcers or blisters
  Associated lower abdominal pain or dysuria
  Adverse effects (redness, irritation or swelling associated with treatment)
  No improvement within 7 days of treatment

Management

Single-dose intravaginal and oral *imidazole* preparations are effective in treating vaginal candidiasis and provide rapid relief from symptoms. Patients find these products very convenient and compliance is higher than with treatments involving several days' use. The patient can be asked whether she prefers a pessary, vaginal cream or oral formulation. Some experts argue that oral antifungals should be reserved for resistant cases. Pharmacists will use their professional judgement together with patient preference in making the decision on treatment.

The pharmacist should make sure that the patient knows how to use the product. An effective way to do this is to show the patient the manufacturer's leaflet instructions. Where external symptoms are also a problem, an *imidazole* cream (*miconazole* or *clotrimazole*) can be useful in addition to the intravaginal or oral product. The cream should be applied twice daily, morning and night.

The *imidazoles* can cause sensitivity reactions but these seem to be rare. However, it is worth checking with the patient whether she has used this type of preparation before and asking about any previous sensitivity problems. Oral *fluconazole* interacts with some drugs:

anticoagulants
oral sulphonylureas
cyclosporin
phenytoin
rifampicin
theophylline.

The effects of single-dose *fluconazole* rather than continuous therapy with the drug in relation to interactions are not clear. Theoretically single-dose use is unlikely to cause problems but pharmacists need to be cautious and take the possibility of interactions into account.

The UK Committee on Safety of Medicines has advised against concomitant administration of oral *fluconazole* with *terfenadine, astemizole* and *cisapride* because the metabolism of these drugs is inhibited by oral *fluconazole* so that the risk of cardiotoxicity is increased. Reported side effects from oral *fluconazole* include nausea, abdominal discomfort, flatulence and diarrhoea. Oral *fluconazole* should not be recommended for nursing mothers because it is excreted in breast milk.

Practical points

Privacy

Patients seeking advice about vaginal symptoms may be embarrassed, fearing that their conversation with the pharmacist will be overheard. It is therefore important to try and ensure privacy. Requests for a named product may be an attempt to avoid discussion. However a careful response is needed to ensure that the product is appropriate.

Treatment of partner

Experts disagree about the need for the partner to be treated if a woman has vaginal candidiasis. An *imidazole* cream can be used twice daily on the glans of the penis, applied under the foreskin. Treatment should be used for 6 days.

'Live' yoghurt

Live yoghurt contains lactobacilli, which are said to alter the vaginal environment, making it more difficult for candida to grow. It has been suggested that women prone to thrush should regularly eat live yoghurt to increase the level of lactobacilli in the gut. The scientific evidence for such claims is lacking, but the recommendation is harmless. Direct application of live yoghurt onto the vulval skin and into the vagina on a tampon has been recommended as a treatment for thrush. This process is messy and some women have reported stinging on application, which is not surprising if the skin is excoriated and sore. Again, it is otherwise harmless, although evidence of effectiveness is lacking.

Prevention

Thrush thrives in a warm environment. Women who are prone to attacks of thrush may find that avoiding nylon underwear and tights and using cotton underwear instead may help prevent future attacks.

The protective lining of the vagina is stripped away by foam baths, soaps and douches and these are best avoided. Vaginal deodorants can themselves cause allergic reactions and should not be used. If the patient wants to use a soap or cleanser, an unperfumed, mild variety is best.

Since candida can be transferred from the bowel when wiping the anus after a bowel movement, wiping from front to back should help to prevent this.

Vaginal thrush in practice

Case 1

Helen Simpson is a student at the local university. She asks one of your assistants for something to treat thrush and is referred to you. You walk with Helen to a quiet area of the shop where your conversation will not be overheard. Initially, Helen is resistant to your involvement, asking why you need to ask 'all these personal questions'. After you have explained that you are required to obtain information before selling these products and that, in any case, you need to be sure that the problem is thrush and not a different infection, she seems happier.

She has not had thrush or any similar symptoms before but described her symptoms to a flatmate who made the 'diagnosis'. The worst symptom is itching, which was particularly severe last night. Helen has noticed small quantities of a creamy-coloured discharge. The vulval skin is sore and red. Helen has a boyfriend, but he hasn't had any symptoms. She is not taking any medicines and does not have any existing illnesses or conditions. Since arriving at the university a few months ago she has not registered with the university's health centre and has therefore come to the pharmacy hoping to buy a treatment.

The pharmacist's view

The key symptoms of itch and creamy vaginal discharge make thrush the most likely candidate here. Helen has no previous history of the condition and, unfortunately, the regulations preclude the recommendation of an intravaginal *imidazole* product or oral *fluconazole* in such a case. An *imidazole* cream would help to ease the itching and soreness of the vulval skin and could also be used by her boyfriend, although he is not experiencing symptoms. However, because external treatment alone is unlikely to prove effective in eradicating the infection, it would be best for Helen to see a doctor.

She would be well advised to register at the university health centre. You can explain to her that she can seek treatment on a 'temporary resident' basis but that it would be best to get proper medical cover.

The doctor's view

The history is very suggestive of thrush and treatment should include an appropriate intravaginal preparation. The case history highlights some of the difficulties of asking personal questions about genitalia and sexual activity. These difficulties are also likely to occur in the doctor's surgery. It is important for the doctor to carefully explore the patient's ideas, understanding, concerns and preconceptions of her condition. Many doctors would prescribe without an examination with such a clear history and only examine and take appropriate microbiology samples if treatment fails.

Eye and Ear Problems

Eye problems: The painful red eye

Conjunctivitis is one cause of a painful red eye. There are other serious causes of painful red eyes and there are several causes of conjunctivitis. Accurate diagnosis of these causes is of vital importance and requires medical knowledge and skills. Referral is therefore essential. Below are notes on some of the causes of painful red eyes.

> **What you should know**
>
> Conjunctivitis
>   Infection
>   Allergy
> Corneal ulcers
> Other causes
>   Iritis
>   Glaucoma

Significance of questions and answers

Conjunctivitis

The term conjunctivitis implies inflammation of the conjunctiva which is a transparent surface covering the white of the eye. It can become inflamed due to infection, allergy or irritation.

Infection

Both bacteria and viruses can cause conjunctivitis. The symptoms are a painful gritty sensation and a discharge. The discharge is sticky and purulent in bacterial infections and more watery in viral. It nearly always affects both eyes. 'Conjunctivitis' occurring in only one eye should alert the doctor to the presence of a foreign body or another condition accounting for the red eye.

Management. Infective conjunctivitis is treated with antibacterial eye drops and ointment. Both bacterial and viral infections are treated in the same way. In viral infections the drops will prevent secondary infections. Quite often it is difficult for the doctor to differentiate between the two types of infection and it safer to assume that it may be bacterial. A typical course of treatment would be to use *chloramphenicol eye drops* every

2 hours for the first 24 hours and then four times daily with *chloramphenicol eye ointment* applied at night for the following week.

Allergy

This produces irritation, discomfort and a watery discharge. It typically occurs in the hay fever season. It is sometimes difficult to differentiate between infection and allergy and so referral is important if there is any doubt.

Management. Sodium cromoglycate eye drops is an effective, safe treatment. Alternatively, decongestant and antihistamine drops can be helpful. Steroid drops are rarely prescribed by the doctor due to their possible side effects of cataract and glaucoma.

Corneal ulcers

These may be due to an infection or a traumatic abrasion. The main symptom is that of pain. There may be surrounding conjunctival inflammation. An abrasion can be caused by wearing contact lenses. Early diagnosis is important as the cornea can become permanently scarred, with loss of sight. If a corneal ulcer is suspected the eye is examined after instilling *fluorescein drops* which will colour and highlight an otherwise invisible ulcer. The cornea is the transparent covering over the front of the eye and early ulcers are not visible.

Management

This is obviously determined by the cause of the ulcer. Specialist referral is invariably required.

Other causes

Iritis

Iritis is inflammation of the iris and surrounding structures. It may occur in association with some forms of arthritis, sarcoidosis or tuberculosis (TB). It may occur as an isolated event with no obvious cause. The inflammation causes pain which is felt more within the eye than the superficial gritty pain of conjunctivitis and there is no discharge. The affected eye is red, the pupil small and possibly irregular. Urgent specialist referral is necessary for accurate diagnosis. Treatment is with topical steroids to reduce inflammation.

Glaucoma

Glaucoma occurs when the pressure of the 'fluids' within the eye becomes abnormally high. This may either happen suddenly or develop slowly and insidiously; two different abnormalities are involved. It is sudden development (acute closed-angle glaucoma) which causes a painful red eye. Emergency hospital referral is necessary in order to prevent permanent loss of sight. The pain of acute glaucoma is severe and may be felt in and around the eye. There may be associated vomiting. As the pressure builds up the cornea swells, becoming hazy, causing impaired vision and a halo appearance around lights. Treatment involves an operation to lower the pressure to prevent it from developing again.

Common ear problems

Although the treatment of common ear problems is straightforward, it does depend upon accurate diagnosis and may require a prescription. It is not always possible to determine the problem from the story. Diagnosis is best made by the doctor, who can examine the ear with an auroscope or otoscope. Referral to the doctor is therefore advisable with ear problems. Ear problems commonly presenting are described below.

What you need to know

Wax
Otitis externa
Otitis media
  Glue ear

Significance of questions and answers

Wax

Symptoms

Wax blocking the ear is one of the commonest causes of temporary deafness. It may also cause discomfort and a sensation that the ear is blocked.

Management

Eardrops. The ear can be unblocked by using eardrops such as olive oil and various proprietary drops. The drops should be warmed before use (ideally to body temperature). With the head inclined, 5 drops should be instilled. A cotton wool plug should be applied to retain the fluid and be kept in for at least an hour or overnight. This procedure should be repeated at least twice a day for 3 days. The use of these drops can worsen the deafness initially and appropriate warning should be given. Cotton wool buds should not be poked into the ear as wax is just pushed further in and it is possible to damage the eardrum.

Syringing ears. If any wax remains despite this treatment then referral to the doctor is advisable so the wax can then be syringed out. The use of drops to soften the wax prior to syringing the ears is in any case recommended to make the procedure more effective.

Otitis externa

Otitis externa is inflammation of the outer ear canal. This is the skin-lined canal which leads into the ear as far as the eardrum. The inflammation is most commonly caused by an infection. Sometimes it is a site of eczema which may become secondarily infected.

Symptoms

The symptoms of otitis externa are usually those of pain and discharge. Referral to the doctor is necessary for accurate diagnosis. It is possible that the same symptoms can arise from a middle ear infection (otitis media) with a perforated eardrum.

Management

Treatment may involve the use of astringent ear drops (e.g. *aluminium acetate*) or antibacterial drops (e.g. *neomycin, polymyxin*) and anti-inflammatory drops (e.g. *hydrocortisone*). In addition any debris or discharge should be removed. This may be achieved by gently syringing, removal under direct vision with a special probe, or the insertion of a ribbon gauze wick soaked in *glycerin* and *icthammol*. Occasionally oral antibiotics are used.

Otitis media

This is an infection of the middle ear compartment. The middle ear lies between the outer ear canal and the inner ear. Between the outer ear and the middle is the eardrum (tympanic membrane). The middle ear is normally an air-containing compartment which is sealed from the outside apart from a small tube (the Eustachian tube) which connects to the back of the throat. Within the middle ear are tiny bones which transmit the sound wave vibrations of the eardrum to the inner ear.

An infection typically starts with a common cold, especially in children, which leads to blockage of the Eustachian tube and fluid formation within the middle ear. The fluid can then be secondarily infected by a bacterial infection.

Symptoms

The symptoms of otitis media are pain and temporary deafness. Sometimes the infection 'takes off' so quickly that the eardrum perforates, releasing the infected fluid. When this occurs a discharge will also be present and be associated with considerable lessening of pain.

Management

As with otitis externa, referral is necessary. Treatment is usually a course of oral antibiotics (e.g. *amoxycillin, penicillin* or *erythromycin*). Sometimes topical or oral decongestants are used in addition to antibiotics. These can be useful if air travel is to be undertaken after such an infection. If the Eustachian tube is still blocked during a flight then pain can be experienced due to the change in air pressure. Decongestants would make this less likely.

Glue ear

Some children who are subject to recurrent otitis media develop 'glue ear'. This occurs because the fluid which forms in the middle ear does not drain out completely. The fluid becomes tenacious and sticky. One method of dealing with this common problem is a minor operation in which the fluid is sucked out through the eardrum. After this it is usual to insert a small grommet into the hole in the drum. The grommet has a small hole in the middle which allows any further fluid forming to drain from the middle ear. The grommet normally falls out within a few months and the small hole in the drum closes over. The effectiveness of this procedure is debatable.

Ear plugs. Some children are advised not to get water into the ear after the insertion of a grommet. One method is to use ear plugs which can be purchased in the pharmacy. Generally, however, this is often unnecessary and bathing and swimming can be undertaken without using plugs, although it is sensible to avoid deep diving as water may enter the middle ear under pressure which will impair hearing and may predispose to infection.

Childhood Conditions

Common childhood rashes

Most childhood rashes are associated with self-limiting viral infections. Some of these rashes fit well-described clinical pictures (e.g. measles) and are described below. Others are more difficult to label. They may appear as short-lived fine flat (macular) or slightly raised (papular) red spots, often on the trunk. The spots blanch with pressure (erythematous). There is usually an associated cold, cough and raised temperature. These relatively minor illnesses occur in the first few years of life and settle without treatment.

What you need to know

Infectious diseases
    Chicken pox
    Measles
    Roseola infantum
    Fifth disease
    German measles
    Meningitis
Rashes which do not blanch

Significance of questions and answers

Chicken pox

This is most common in children under 10 years old. It can occur in adults but is unusual. The incubation time (i.e. time between contact and development of rash) is usually about 2 weeks (11–21 days). Sometimes the rash is preceded by a day or so of feeling unwell with a temperature. The rash is characteristic and only difficult to diagnose when very few spots are present. Typically it starts with small red lumps which rapidly develop into minute blisters (vesicles). The vesicles then burst, forming crusted spots over the next few days. The spots mainly occur on the trunk and face but may involve the mucous membranes of the mouth. They tend to come out in crops for up to 5 days. The rash is often irritant. Once the spots have all formed crusts, the individual is no longer contagious. The whole infection is usually over within a week but it may be longer and more severe in adults.

The symptoms may be eased with *calamine* lotion and *paracetamol* if a high temperature is present. Warm salt baths may be comforting.

Measles
This is now a less common infection in the more developed countries. Since 1968 all infants in the UK have been routinely offered the measles vaccine at about 13 months old. This has now been superseded by the introduction of MMR, a combined measles, mumps and rubella vaccine, between the ages of 1 and 2 years. Measles has an incubation period of about 10 days. The measles rash is preceded by 3–4 days of illness with cold symptoms, cough, conjunctivitis and fever. After the first 2 days of this prodromal phase small white spots (Koplik spots), like grains of salt, can be seen on the inner cheek and gums. The measles rash then follows. It starts behind the ears, spreading to the face and trunk. The spots are small red patches (macules) which will blanch if pressed. Sometimes there are so many spots that they merge together to form large red areas.

Complications
At present there are about 10 deaths a year in England and Wales from encephalitis (inflammation of the brain) which is a rare complication of measles. In most cases the rash fades after 3 days, at which time the fever also subsides. If, however, the fever persists, the cough becomes worse or there is difficulty in breathing or earache, then medical attention should be sought.

Roseola infantum
This is a viral infection occurring most commonly in the first year of life (but also between 3 months and 4 years of age). It can be confused with a mild attack of measles. There is a prodromal period of 3–4 days of fever followed by a rash similar to measles but which is mainly confined to the chest and abdomen. Once the rash appears there is usually an improvement in symptoms, in contrast to measles and it only lasts about 24 hours.

Fifth disease (erythema infectiosum)
This is another viral infection which usually affects children. It does not often cause systemic upset but may cause fever, headache and painful joints. The rash characteristically starts on the face. It gives an appearance that the cheeks have been slapped or that the child has been out in a cold wind. The rash then appears on the limbs and trunk as small red spots which blanch with pressure. The infection is usually short-lived.

German measles (rubella)

This viral infection is generally very mild, its main significance being the problems caused to the foetus if a pregnant mother develops the infection in early pregnancy. The rash is preceded by mild catarrhal symptoms and enlargement of glands at the back of the neck. It usually starts on the face and spreads to the trunk and limbs. The spots are very fine and red. They blanch with pressure. They do not become confluent as in measles. In adults rubella may be associated with painful joints. The rubella rash lasts 3–5 days.

Meningitis

In very rare situations a rash may be associated with meningococcal septicaemia. This very serious infection causes meningitis. It usually presents with flu-like symptoms which progress to vomiting, headache and neck stiffness. There may be an associated rash present which appears as small widespread bruises (very small bruises are called petechiae, larger ones ecchymoses). Bruises do not blanch with pressure. This condition requires emergency medical help.

Rashes which do not blanch

As a general rule all rashes which do not blanch when pressed ought to be referred to a doctor. These rashes are caused by blood leaking out of a capillary, which may be caused by a blood disorder. It could be the first sign of leukaemia.

> **When to refer**
>
> Suspected meningitis
>   Flu-like symptoms
>   Vomiting
>   Headache
>   Neck stiffness
>   Rash
>   Small widespread bruises which do not blanch when pressed
> Rashes which do not blanch when pressed.

Management

The itching caused by childhood rashes such as chicken pox can be intense and the pharmacist is in a good position to offer an antipruritic cream, ointment or lotion. *Aqueous calamine cream* is an excellent preparation to soothe itchy skin and its effectiveness can be increased further by adding 1% menthol. The addition of *menthol* provides an antipruritic and cooling effect which can be very comforting for irritated skin. *Calamine lotion* is an effective antipruritic and leaves a soothing layer of powder on the skin once the liquid vehicle has evaporated. Some patients find *calamine lotion* messy to use. *Aqueous calamine cream* is non-greasy and easily absorbed and is preferred by many patients.

If itching is very severe, a systemic antihistamine such as *promethazine* can be effective in providing relief. Such treatment would be likely to make the child drowsy but may be useful at night-time.

Napkin rash

Most babies will have napkin (nappy) rash at some stage during their infancy. Contributory factors include contact of urine and faeces with the skin, wetness and maceration of skin due to infrequent nappy changes and inadequate skin care. Advice from the pharmacist is important in both treating and preventing recurrence of the problem.

What you need to know

Nature and location of rash
Severity
   Broken skin
   Signs of infection
Duration
Previous history
Other symptoms
Precipitating factors
   Skin care and hygiene
Medication

Significance of questions and answers

Nature and location of rash

Nappy rash, sometimes called napkin dermatitis, appears as an erythematous rash on the buttock area. Other areas of the body are not involved, in contrast to infantile seborrheic dermatitis, where the scalp may also be affected (cradle cap). In infantile eczema, involvement of other body areas usually occurs. Initial treatment of nappy rash would be the same in each case.

Severity

In general, if the skin is unbroken and there are no signs of secondary bacterial infection treatment may be considered. The presence of bacterial infection would be signified by weeping or yellow crusting. Secondary fungal infection is common in napkin dermatitis and the presence of satellite papules—small red lesions near the perimeter of the affected area—would indicate such an infection.

Referral to the doctor would be advisable if bacterial infection were suspected, since topical or systemic antibiotics might be needed.

Secondary fungal infection could be treated by the pharmacist using one of the *imidazole* topical antifungal preparations which are available.

Duration

If the condition had been present for longer than 2 weeks, the pharmacist might decide that referral to the doctor would be the best option, depending on the nature and severity of the rash.

Previous history

The pharmacist should establish whether the problem has occurred before and, if so, what action was taken; for example, treatment with over-the-counter (OTC) products.

Other symptoms

Napkin dermatitis sometimes occurs during or after a bout of diarrhoea, when the perianal skin can become reddened and sore. The pharmacist should therefore enquire about current or recent incidence of diarrhoea. Diarrhoea may occur as a side effect of antibiotic therapy and this may be the cause. Sometimes thrush in the nappy area may be associated with oral thrush which causes a sore mouth or throat (see p. 259). If this is suspected, referral to the doctor is advisable.

Precipitating factors

Skin care and hygiene

At one time, napkin dermatitis was thought to be a simple irritant dermatitis due to ammonia, produced as a breakdown product of urine in soiled nappies, however, other factors are now known to play a part in the development of the condition. These include irritant substances in urine and faeces; sensitivity reactions to detergents and antiseptics left in terry nappies after inadequate rinsing; and sensitivity reactions to ingredients in some topical preparations, for example, *lanolin*. However, the major factor thought to influence the incidence of nappy rash is the constant wetting and re-wetting of the skin when left in contact with soiled nappies. Maceration of the skin ensues, leading to enhanced penetration of irritant substances through the skin and the breakdown of the skin. The wearing of occlusive plastic pants exacerbates this effect. Frequent changes of nappy together with good nappy-changing routine and hygiene are essential (see *Practical points* below).

Medication

The identity and effectiveness of any preparations used for the current or any previous episode, either prescribed or purchased OTC, should be ascertained by the pharmacist. The possibility of a sensitivity reaction to an ingredient in a topical product already tried should be considered by the pharmacist, especially if the rash has worsened.

When to refer

Broken skin, severe rash
Signs of infection
Other body areas affected

Treatment timescale

A baby with nappy rash which does not respond to skin care and OTC treatment within a week should be seen by the doctor.

Management

Treatment of napkin dermatitis and the prevention of further episodes can be achieved by a combination of OTC treatment and advice on care of the skin in the nappy area.

Emollient preparations

Emollient preparations are the mainstay of treatment. The inclusion of a water repellent such as *dimethicone* may be useful (e.g. in *dimethicone cream BP*). Such preparations can help to protect the skin against water. The choice of individual preparation may sometimes depend on customer preference and many preparations are equally effective. Most pharmacists will have a particular favourite which they usually recommend. Some of the ingredients included in preparations for the treatment and prevention of nappy rash and their uses are described below.

Zinc

Zinc acts as a soothing agent.

Lanolin

Lanolin emollient hydrates the skin. It can sometimes cause sensitivity reactions, although the high grades of purified *lanolin* used in many of today's products should reduce the problem.

Castor oil/cod liver oil

These provide a water-resistant layer on the skin.

Antibacterials (e.g. *chlorhexidine gluconate*)

These may be useful in reducing the numbers of bacteria on the skin. Some antibacterials have been reported to produce sensitivity reactions.

Antifungals

Secondary infection with candida is common in napkin dermatitis and the *imidazole* antifungals would be effective. *Miconazole* or *clotrimazole* applied twice daily could be recommended by the pharmacist with advice to consult the doctor if the rash did not improve within 5 days. If an antifungal cream is advised, treatment should be continued for 4 or 5 days after the symptoms have apparently cleared. An emollient cream or ointment can still be applied over the antifungal product.

Hydrocortisone

Prescription only medicine (POM)

Hydrocortisone cream or *ointment* cannot be sold by pharmacists for the treatment of nappy rash because its use OTC is restricted to children aged over 10 years. Topical steroids are effective treatments for napkin dermatitis and other preparations containing steroids may well be prescribed by the doctor for this purpose. Pharmacists can give valuable advice about the correct method of use.

Method of use

First, the preparation should be applied thinly and sparingly: the pharmacist can reassure the parents that only a small amount is needed for effectiveness. Second, the absorption of corticosteroids from topical vehicles is increased when the skin is occluded by the wearing of plastic pants. Systemic side-effects have occasionally occured as a result of large quantities of topical steroids being applied followed by occlusion under waterproof pants. The more potent the steroid, the higher the chance such adverse effects will be produced. Parents should be reminded that if the condition does not respond quickly to treatment (within 10 days) further advice should be sought from the doctor.

Practical points

1 Nappies should be changed as frequently as necessary. Babies up to 3 months old may pass urine as many as 12 times a day.

2 Nappies should be left off wherever possible so that air is able to circulate around the skin, helping the affected skin to become and remain dry. Lying the baby on a terry nappy or towel with a waterproof sheet underneath will prevent the soiling of furniture or bedding.

3 Providing terry nappies are changed sufficiently often, rinsed

thoroughly after washing to remove traces of detergent and used with a good quality nappy liner, there is no reason to abandon them for disposables. The technology of water-absorbent materials has advanced considerably in recent years and current disposable nappies are able to keep the skin in the nappy area very dry. However, disposable nappies must still be changed regularly. There is no clear case to recommend one type of nappy over the other—skin care and regular changing remain the most important factors (see 6 below).

4 Waterproof pants create an occlusive barrier which prevents the evaporation of moisture and can worsen napkin dermatitis. If such garments are to be used at all, they should only be used for short periods of time.

5 Washing routine for terry nappies is important. If a sanitizing solution is used to soak the nappies, thorough rinsing is needed before washing. The nappies should be rinsed well after washing to ensure that no chemicals are left in the fabric which might irritate the baby's skin. Towelling nappies may be bleached occasionally before washing, but thorough rinsing is essential.

6 At each nappy change the skin should be cleansed thoroughly by washing with warm water or using a proprietary lotion or wipes. The skin should then be carefully and thoroughly dried. The use of talcum powder can be helpful, but the clumping of powder can sometimes cause further irritation. Talcum powder should always be applied to dry skin and should be dusted lightly over the nappy area. The regular use of an emollient cream or ointment, applied to clean dry skin, can help to protect the skin against irritant substances.

Napkin rash in practice

Case 1

Jane Simmonds, a young mother, asks you to recommend a good cream for her baby daughter's nappy rash. The baby (Sarah) is 3 months old and Mrs Simmonds tells you that the buttocks are covered in a red rash. The skin is not broken and there is no weeping or yellow matter present. On further questioning, you find that the rash is also affecting the upper back and neck and there are signs of its appearance around the wrists. The rash seems to be itchy, as Sarah keeps trying to scratch the affected areas. Mrs Simmonds uses disposable nappies, which she changes frequently and *zinc and castor oil cream* is applied at each nappy change, after cleansing the skin. The baby has no other symptoms and is not taking any medicines.

The pharmacist's view

Mrs Simmonds' nappy-changing and skin-care routine seems to be adequate, but the baby has nappy rash and the rash affects other areas of the body. It is possible that Sarah has infantile eczema and referral to the doctor would be the best course of action.

The doctor's view

It is quite likely that Sarah does have eczema, which could be the cause of her nappy rash. It is also possible that an eczematous rash can be complicated by a secondary infection. Referral to the doctor or health visitor for further assessment would be wise. Such skin problems can be an emotive topic and it is important that Mrs Simmonds should be given an opportunity to air her understanding of, and concerns about, the problem and in return that the doctor offers an appropriate explanation. The management would be to reinforce all the above practical points and possibly prescribe a weak topical steroid such as 1% *hydrocortisone* with or without an antifungal or antibacterial agent.

Case 2

Mrs Lesley Tibbs is worried about her baby son's nappy rash, which she tells you seems to have appeared over the last few days. The skin is quite red and sore-looking and she has been using a proprietary cream, but the rash seems to be even worse. The baby has never had nappy rash before and is about 5 months old. Mrs Tibbs is using towelling nappies which she soaks in a proprietary solution before washing them in an automatic washing machine. She has recently changed the washing powder she uses, on a friend's recommendation. The rash affects only the napkin area and the baby has no other symptoms.

The pharmacist's view

The history gives two clues to the possible cause of the problem. This baby has not had nappy rash before and this episode has coincided with a change in detergent, so it is possible that a sensitivity reaction is occuring due to residues of detergent remaining in the nappies after washing. The second factor is the cream which Mrs Tibbs has been using to treat the problem, with no success. The ingredients of the product should be carefully considered by the pharmacist to see if any might be potential sensitizers, for example *lanolin* or *chlorhexidine gluconate*.

Initial advice to Mrs Tibbs might be to revert to her original detergent and to use a different treatment. Advice on nappy-changing routine could be given and if the rash had not started to resolve within a week, or had become worse, referral to the doctor should be indicated.

The doctor's view

The advice given by the pharmacist should clear the problem up quickly. It would be quite reasonable to refer Mrs Tibbs and her baby to the health visitor for further advice if the rash did not settle down.

Head lice

Head lice infection is common in young children. Effective treatments are available, but treatment failure may occur if products are not used correctly. It is therefore important for the pharmacist to explain how products should be used, since more patients are now being directed to pharmacies to obtain treatment. The pharmacist has a valuable health education role in explaining how to check children's hair for lice and in discouraging prophylactic use of insecticides. Parents are often embarrassed to seek advice, particularly if the child has head lice. Pharmacists can reassure parents that the condition is common and does not in any way indicate a lack of hygiene. The term 'infection' is preferred to 'infestation' by some pharmacists when talking to parents because of the unpleasant image associated with infestation.

What you need to know
Age
Child, adult
Signs of infection
Live lice
Checking for infection
Nits
Scalp itching
Previous infection
Medication
Treatments used

Significance of questions and answers

Age
Head lice infection is most commonly found in children, particularly at around 4–5 years old. Older children and adults seem to be less prone to infection. Adult women occasionally become infected, but head lice infection is rare in adult men because as men lose hair through male pattern baldness the scalp offers less shelter to lice.

Signs of infection
Unless infection has been confirmed by a nurse or doctor who has

inspected the scalp, the pharmacist should check whether any inspection has been made to confirm the presence of head lice. Parents often worry that their children may catch lice and wish the pharmacist to recommend prophylactic treatment. Insecticides should never be used prophylactically, since this may accelerate resistance. Treatment should be reserved for infected heads. However a louse repellent is now available (see p. 253).

Checking for infection

Parents can easily check for infection by combing the child's hair over a piece of white or light-coloured paper, using a fine-toothed comb. The hair should be damp or wet to make the combing process easier and less painful. Also dry hair can produce static that causes lice to be repelled from the comb, making detection less likely. If live lice are present, some will be combed out of the hair and onto the paper, where they will be seen as small greyish-white or brown-coloured specks. Cast shells are discarded as the louse grows and appear yellowish in colour. Louse faeces may be seen as small blackish specks on pillows and collars. The hair at the nape of the neck and behind the ears should be thoroughly checked. These spots are preferred by lice because they are warm and relatively sheltered. Such a check should be carried out regularly, say once a week, and perhaps more often when infection is known to have occurred in other children at school or playgroup.

Nits

The presence of empty egg shells—the cream- or white-coloured 'nits' attached to the hair shafts—is not necessarily evidence of current infection unless live lice are also found. Parents sometimes think that treatment has failed because nits can still be seen in the hair. It is therefore important for the pharmacist to explain that the empty shells are firmly glued to the hair shaft and will not be removed by the lotion used in treatment. A fine-toothed comb can be used to remove the nits after treatment.

Itching

Contrary to popular belief itching is not experienced by everyone with a head lice infection. In fact as few as one in five cases present with itching, perhaps because detection occurs at an earlier stage than used to be the case. Where it occurs, itching of the scalp is an allergic response to the saliva of the lice, which is injected into the scalp in small amounts each time the lice feed. Sensitization does not occur immediately and it may take weeks for itching to develop. It has been estimated that thousands of bites from the lice are required before the reaction develops.

The absence of itching does not mean that infection has not occurred. In someone who has previously been infected and becomes reinfected, itching may quickly begin again.

Previous infection

The pharmacist should establish whether the child has been infected before. In particular, it is important to know whether there has been a recent infection, as reinfection may have occurred from other family members if the whole family was not treated at the same time. Head-to-head contact, between family members and also among young children while playing, is responsible for the transmission of head lice from one host to the next. The pharmacist could ask whether the parent was aware of any contact with infected children, for example, if there is currently a problem with head lice at the child's school.

Medication

While it is possible that treatment failure may occur, this is unlikely if a recommended insecticide has been used (see *Management* section) and the product has been used correctly. Careful questioning will be needed to determine whether treatment failure has occurred. The identity of any treatment used and its method of use should be elicited.

Management

Local policy

Having established that infection is present, the pharmacist can go on to recommend an appropriate treatment. Insecticide policies were set up throughout the country to try and prevent the development of resistance. Policies still exist in many parts of the country and are usually set up on a National Health Service (NHS) Health Authority basis. Three types of insecticide, *malathion, carbaryl* and the pyrethroids are used on a rotational basis. *Carbaryl* is now a prescription only medicine (POM) in the UK whereas *malathion* and the pyrethroids can be sold over the counter (OTC).

The Pharmaceutical Adviser or Drug Information Unit will be able to provide information on whether a policy exists and which insecticide is currently in use. If patients ask for a head lice treatment by name and the product does not contain the recommended insecticide, pharmacists can explain about the rotational policy and try to persuade the patient to accept an approved product.

Informing doctors about the local policy is important and pharmacists could let local practices know when a change occurs and remind them of the current recommendations. This should minimize the possibility of conflicting advice and information being given.

Pharmacists can also work with health visitors to communicate with schools in the area and ensure the accuracy and currency of information given to parents and children. If there is no formal rotational policy, 'mosaic' prescribing is sometimes advised, where the doctor or pharmacist recommend different insecticides sequentially to each presenting case.

There is still a stigma attached to head lice infection and many parents feel ashamed if their children become infected, feeling that infection must be a sign of poor hygiene. Of course this is not so and pharmacists can reassure their customers that head lice infection is not only extremely common, but equally likely to occur in clean hair as in dirty hair. Head-to-head contact means that lice are easily transferred from one person to the next.

Malathion, permethrin and phenothrin

These can be recommended OTC. It is generally recommended that all members of the family should be treated at the same time to prevent reinfection from another family member. Another approach is to treat only those in whom infection has been confirmed and to check the hair of all family members on a regular basis to look for infection. However, the latter requires a high level of motivation. Checking the hair by combing over white paper and visual inspection should confirm who is infected. Contact tracing is important to track the source of the infection and also to identify who might have become infected.

Family-sized treatment packs are available for some products. The pharmacist can advise doctors about the amount of lotion necessary to treat each person—this is sometimes underestimated by prescribers and should be 50–55 ml per person as a minimum. Using too little treatment has been a cause of treatment failure in the past, necessitating repeated treatment.

Carbaryl

Carbaryl is now available only on prescription in the UK. Data from animal studies indicated the possibility of carcinogenicity and the theoretical risk to humans led to the change in legal classification in 1996.

Lotion or shampoo?

Lotions and cream rinse formulations are the preferred treatment for head lice. A lotion is applied to the scalp and the hair left to dry. The insecticide is therefore in contact with the hair for a long period of time and at a high concentration. In contrast, a shampoo is diluted by adding water, so that the concentration of insecticide is low. After shampooing the hair is rinsed, so that the insecticide is in contact with the scalp for only a short time. Because several applications of shampoo are needed, compliance may not be achieved and treatment failure can result.

Alcoholic and aqueous lotions

Malathion and *carbaryl* are available as alcoholic and aqueous lotions. Alcohol-based formulations are generally useful but are not suitable for all patients because they can cause two types of problem. First, alcohol can cause stinging when applied to scalps with skin broken as a result of scratching. Babies and other patients with eczema affecting the scalp may also experience stinging. Second, in patients with asthma it is thought that alcohol-based lotions are best avoided, as the evaporating alcohol might irritate the lungs and cause wheezing, perhaps even precipitating an attack of asthma. Such reactions are likely to be extremely rare, but caution is still advised.

If available, aqueous lotions are to be preferred for these patients and also for small children, to avoid alcoholic fumes.

Indications for shampoo

Shampoos are generally not to be recommended. Their clinical effectiveness is less than lotion and cream rinse formulations. In the past shampoos were an alternative where alcoholic lotions were not suitable. However aqueous versions of treatments are now available.

Method of use and advice

Malathion and carbaryl

Lotions. These should be rubbed gently into dry hair and care should be taken to ensure that the scalp is thoroughly covered. The most effective method of application is to sequentially part sections of the hair and then apply a few drops of the treatment, spreading it along the parting, into the surrounding scalp and along the hair. Approximately 50–55 ml of lotion should be sufficient for one application although people with very thick or long hair may need more. A towel or cloth can be placed over the eyes and face to protect them from the lotion. When applying the product, particular attention should be paid to the areas at the nape of the neck and behind the ears, where lice are often found. The hair should then be left to dry naturally. Hair driers or other heat sources should not be used with carbaryl and malathion because both are inactivated by heat. In addition, where an alcoholic lotion is used, the hair should be kept away from fire and naked flames.

The hair can be shampooed 2 hours after applying the lotion, but leaving the lotion in contact with the hair for 12 hours or longer can help to produce a residual effect from the insecticide.

A repeat application is now advised 7 days after the initial treatment. This second application will kill any lice which have emerged from eggs in the meantime.

Malathion and carbaryl shampoos. These are rarely used and are included here only for completeness. The hair should be shampooed with the insecticidal product and rinsed, then the application should be repeated, leaving the shampoo on the hair for 5 minutes before rinsing off. Warm rather than hot water should be used to minimize the chances of the insecticide being inactivated. Following the first treatment, the product should be used twice more, at 3-day intervals. This regime for shampoos is necessary because the incubation period for head lice is 7–10 days. While no new eggs would be laid after the first application of shampoo, there remains the possibility that some live eggs would not have been killed and so may hatch out, hence the need for two further applications.

Permethrin and phenothrin lotions

Permethrin. This is formulated as a cream rinse containing 20% alcohol. The hair should first be washed, rinsed and towel dried (if the hair is too wet, the cream rinse will not adhere properly). The cream rinse should be massaged well into the towel-dried hair to soak both hair and scalp, and then left on for 10 minutes before rinsing thoroughly with water and drying as normal. A residual effect may last for up to 6 weeks. Permethrin is not inactivated by chlorine in swimming pools.

Phenothrin. This is formulated as a lotion containing approximately 70% alcohol. The lotion is sprinkled onto dry hair and rubbed gently until hair and scalp are soaked. The hair is then left to dry naturally. The manufacturers say that after 2 hours the hair can be shampooed normally. *Phenothrin* is not inactivated by chlorine in swimming pools.

Removing eggs and nits

After using a lotion or shampoo, a fine-toothed dust comb can be used to remove the eggs and empty shells (nits), which will have remained glued to the hair shafts. Combing is best done next time the hair is washed, while the hair is wet.

Residual effect

A residual effect from insecticides can occur after the use of lotions, but not shampoos. The effect takes several hours of contact to develop when using *carbaryl* and *malathion* and the level of residual action varies from person to person. Once established, the effect may last for several weeks. In the case of *carbaryl* and *malathion*, contact with chlorinated water during swimming will reduce any residual effect, as will the application of heat via hairdryers.

Repellents

A head louse repellent product containing *piperonal* is available in the UK. The chemical affects the head louse's perception of temperature such that the hair appears cool. The louse is unlikely to transfer to such a head since lice need warm temperatures. The use of repellents may help to reduce the inappropriate use of insecticides for the 'prevention' of head lice infection. A repellent can be particularly useful in preventing reinfection and spread before the source of the infection is identified.

Head lice in practice

Case 1

A young mother, who often comes into your pharmacy to ask advice and buy medicines for her children, asks for a product to prevent head lice. Her children have not got head lice but she wants to use a soap or shampoo 'just to be on the safe side'. On questioning, you find out that the children are aged 5 and 7 and that there are no signs of infection such as itching scalps. The children's heads have not been checked for lice—she is not sure how to go about making such a check. There has not been any communication from the children's school to indicate that head lice is a current problem at the school. This lady explains that she is very hygiene conscious and would hate her children to get nits.

The pharmacist's view

Insecticides should never be recommended unless there is evidence of infection. From what this mother has said it seems unlikely that her children have head lice and there is no evidence of a current problem at school. The pharmacist can therefore reassure her that infection is unlikely. In cases such as this where parents with their children's interest at heart seek to use insecticides to prevent infection, careful explanation from the pharmacist is required. First, the parent can be reassured that head lice and hygiene have absolutely nothing to do with each other and that lice actually prefer clean heads. Head lice are easily transferred from one head to another, particularly among schoolchildren. It is important to stress that insecticide lotions or shampoos will be ineffective in preventing infection and may even contribute to the development of resistant lice. The ritual head-washing with insecticidal soap which was a feature of some parents' own childhood was both unnecessary and ineffective.

The pharmacist can then explain how to make weekly checks for lice using a fine-toothed comb and a light-coloured sheet of paper. If any signs are found this woman should return to the pharmacy, at which time the pharmacist will recommend an insecticide. In the meantime, if the mother is keen to do something more active, a repellent product could be recommended.

The doctor's view

The advice given by the pharmacist is very helpful. It would have certainly been a lot quicker and more convenient, but inappropriate, to have sold the mother a lotion or shampoo. Hopefully the information given by the pharmacist will allay her anxiety regarding hygiene and lice. This demonstrates an important role of health education that can be provided in the pharmacy.

Threadworms

Infection with threadworms (*Enterobius vermicularis*) is common in young children and parents may seek advice from the pharmacist. As with head lice infections, many parents feel embarrassed about discussing threadworms and feel ashamed that their child is infected. Pharmacists can give reassurance that this is a commonly seen problem. In addition to recommending over-the-counter (OTC) anthelmintic treatment, it is essential that advice is given about hygiene measures to prevent reinfection.

What you need to know
Age
Signs of infection
Perianal itching
Appearance of worms
Other symptoms
Duration
Recent travel abroad
Other family members affected
Medication

Significance of questions and answers

Age
Threadworm infection is very common in schoolchildren.

Signs of infection
The first sign that parents notice is usually that the child is scratching his or her bottom. Perianal itching is a classic symptom of threadworm infection and is caused by an allergic reaction to the substances in and surrounding the worms' eggs, which are laid around the anus. Sensitization takes a while to develop so in someone infected for the first time itching will not necessarily occur.

Itching is worse at night, because at that time the female worms emerge from the anus to lay their eggs on the surrounding skin. The eggs are secreted together with a sticky irritant fluid onto the perianal skin. Persistent scratching may lead to secondary bacterial infection. If the perianal skin is broken and there are signs of weeping, referral to the doctor for antibiotic treatment would be advisable.

Loss of sleep due to itching may lead to tiredness and irritability during the day.

Itching without the confirmatory sighting of threadworms may be due to other causes, such as an allergic or irritant dermatitis caused by soaps or topical treatments used to treat the itching. In some patients, scabies or fungal infection may produce perianal itching.

Appearance of worms

The worms themselves can be easily seen in the faeces as white or cream-coloured thread-like objects, about 10 mm in length and less than half a millimetre in width. Males are smaller than females. The worms can survive outside the body for a short time and hence may be seen to be moving. Sometimes the worms may be seen protruding from the anus itself.

Other symptoms

In severe cases of infection, diarrhoea may be present and, in girls, vaginal itch.

Duration

If a threadworm infection is identified, the pharmacist needs to know how long the symptoms have been present and to consider this information in the light of any treatments tried.

Recent travel abroad

If any infection other than threadworm is suspected, patients should be referred to their doctor for further investigation. If the person has recently travelled abroad, this information should be passed on to the doctor so that other types of worm can be considered.

Other family members

The pharmacist should enquire whether any other member of the family is experiencing the same symptoms. However, the absence of perianal itching and threadworms in the faeces does not mean that the person is not infected; it is important to remember that during the early stages, these symptoms may not occur.

Medication

The pharmacist should enquire about the identity of any treatment tried already to treat the symptoms. For any anthelmintic agent, correct use is essential if treatment is to be successful. The pharmacist should therefore also ask how the treatment was used, in order to establish whether treatment failure might be due to incorrect use.

Management

When recommending treatment for threadworms, it is important that the pharmacist emphasizes how and when the treatment is to be used. In addition, advice about preventing recurrence can be given, as described under *Practical points* below. If symptoms do not remit after correct use of an appropriate preparation, patients should see their doctor.

Mebendazole

Mebendazole is the preferred treatment for threadworms. *Mebendazole* is an effective, single-dose treatment against threadworm which is also active against whipworm, roundworm and hookworm. Compliance with therapy is high because of the single dose. The drug is formulated as a single tablet, which can be given to children aged 2 years and over. The dose is one tablet for children and adults. Reinfection is common and a second dose can be given after 2–3 weeks. Occasionally abdominal pain and diarrhoea may occur as side effects. *Mebendazole* is not recommended for pregnant women.

Piperazine

Piperazine is effective against threadworm and roundworm. It is available in granular form in sachets and also as an elixir; the pharmacist can select the more appropriate formulation for the patient. The mode of action of *piperazine* seems to be paralysis of the threadworms in the gut. The incorporation of a laxative (*senna*) in the sachet preparation helps to ensure that the paralysed worms are then expelled with the faeces.

Instructions

The instructions for use must be followed exactly. For the sachet version, one dose is followed by a another 2 weeks later. The elixir is given daily for 7 days, with a further 7 days' treatment if required. Such repeat dosing is designed to destroy any worms which might have hatched and developed after the first dose of drug. For young children, the sachet formulation may be the most acceptable, since added to water it forms a fruit-flavoured drink. Only two doses are required.

Side effects
Side effects of *piperazine* include nausea, vomiting, diarrhoea and colic but these are uncommon. Adverse effects on the central nervous system (CNS) include headaches and dizziness but these are rare.

Contra-indications
Piperazine can be recommended OTC for children from 1 year of age onwards. It should not be recommended for pregnant women because, although a direct causal relationship has not been established, some cases of foetal malformations have been reported. Its use is contra-indicated in epileptic patients since it has been shown to have the potential to induce fits in patients with *grand mal* epilepsy. *Piperazine* may also potentiate extrapyramidal side effects of *chlorpromazine* and should not be recommended for patients on neuroleptic therapy. Where impairment of renal function is present, *piperazine* should not be used.

In some European countries, *piperazine* has been removed from the market because of concern about adverse effects.

Practical points
1 Parents are often anxious and ashamed that their child has a threadworm infection, thinking that lack of hygiene is responsible. The pharmacist can reassure parents that threadworm infection is extremely common and that any child can become infected; infection does not signify a lack of care and attention.
2 All family members should be treated at the same time, even if only one has been shown to have threadworms. This is because other members may be in the early stages of infection and thus asymptomatic. If this policy is not followed, reinfection may occur.
3 Transmission of, and reinfection by, threadworms can be prevented by the following practical measures.
   (a) Cutting fingernails short to prevent large numbers of eggs being transmitted. Hands should be washed and nails brushed after going to the toilet and before preparing or eating food, since hand to mouth transfer of eggs is common. Eggs may be transmitted from the fingers while eating food, or onto the surface of food during preparation. Eggs remain viable for up to a week.
   (b) The wearing of pyjamas by children to reduce the scratching of bare skin during the night. Underpants can be worn under pyjama bottoms.
   (c) Affected family members having a bath or shower each morning to wash away the eggs which were laid during the previous night.

Oral thrush

Thrush (candidosis) is a fungal infection which occurs commonly in the mouth (oral thrush), in the nappy area in babies and in the vagina (see p. 218). Oral thrush in babies can be treated by the pharmacist.

Significance of questions and answers

Age

Oral thrush is most common in babies, particularly in the first few weeks of life. Often, the infection is passed on by the mother during childbirth. In older children and adults, oral thrush is rarer, but may occur after antibiotic or inhaled steroid treatment (see *Medication* section below). In this older group it may also be a sign of immunosuppression and referral to the doctor is advisable.

Affected areas

Oral thrush affects the surface of the tongue and the insides of the cheeks.

Appearance

Oral thrush

When candidal infection involves mucosal surfaces, white patches known as 'plaques' are formed which resemble milk curds; indeed, they may be confused with the latter by mothers when oral thrush occurs in babies. The distinguishing feature of plaques due to candida is that they are not so easily removed from the mucosa and when the surface of the plaque is scraped away, a sore and reddened area of mucosa will be seen underneath, which may sometimes bleed.

Napkin rash

In the napkin (nappy) area, candidal infection presents differently, with characteristic red papules on the outer edge of the area of nappy rash, so-called 'satellite papules'. Another feature is that the skin in the skin folds is nearly always affected. Candidal infection is now thought to be an important factor in the development of nappy rash (see p. 244).

Previous history

In babies recurrent infection is uncommon, although it may sometimes occur following reinfection from the mother's nipples during breastfeeding, or from inadequately sterilized bottle teats in bottle-fed babies.

Patients who experience recurrent infections should be referred to their doctor for further investigation.

Human immunodeficiency virus (HIV) infection

Persistence of oral thrush and/or thrush of the nappy area after the neonatal period may be the first sign of HIV infection.

Medication

Antibiotics

Some drugs predispose to the development of thrush. For example, broad-spectrum antibiotic therapy can wipe out the normal bacterial flora, allowing the overgrowth of fungal infection. It would be useful to establish whether the patient has recently taken a course of antibiotics.

Immunosuppressives

Any drug which suppresses the immune system will reduce resistance to infection and immunocompromised patients are more likely to get thrush. Cytotoxic therapy and steroids predispose to thrush. Patients using inhaled steroids for asthma are prone to oral thrush because steroid is deposited at the back of the throat during inhalation, especially if inhaler technique is poor. Rinsing the throat with water after using the inhaler may be helpful.

The pharmacist should identify any treatment already tried to treat the problem. In a patient with recurrent thrush it would be worth enquiring about previously prescribed therapy and its success.

When to refer

Recurrent infection
All except babies
Failed medication

Treatment timescale

Oral thrush should respond to treatment quickly. If the symptoms have not cleared up within a week, patients should see their doctor.

Management

Antifungal agents

Miconazole

The only specially formulated product currently available for sale over the counter (OTC) to treat oral thrush is *miconazole gel*. Preparations containing *nystatin* are also effective treatments, but are restricted to prescription only status.

Miconazole gel is an orange-flavoured product which should be applied to the plaques using a clean finger four times daily after food in adults and children over 6 years old and twice daily in younger children and infants. For young babies, the gel can be applied directly to the lesions using a cotton bud or the handle of a teaspoon. The gel should be retained in the mouth for as long as possible.

Treatment should be continued for 2 clear days after the symptoms have apparently gone, to ensure that all infection is eradicated.

Interaction. Miconazole gel should not be recommended for patients taking anticoagulants. There is evidence of an interaction with *warfarin* leading to an increase in bleeding time.

Practical points

Oral thrush and nappy rash

If a baby has oral thrush, the pharmacist should check whether nappy rash is also present. Where both oral thrush and candidal involvement in nappy rash occur, both should be treated at the same time. An antifungal cream containing *miconazole* or *clotrimazole* can be used for the nappy area.

Breastfeeding

Where the mother is breastfeeding, a small amount of *miconazole* gel applied to the nipples will eradicate any fungus present. For bottle-fed babies, particular care should be taken to sterilize bottles and teats.

Oral thrush in practice

Case 1

Helen Jones, a young mother, brings her daughter Jane to see you. Ms Jones wants you to recommend something for Jane's mouth, which has white patches on the tongue and inside the cheeks. Jane is 8 years old and is not currently taking any medicines. She has not recently had any antibiotics or other prescribed medicines. Jane does not have any other symptoms.

The pharmacist's view

Jane should be referred to her doctor, since thrush is rare in children other than infants. There is no apparent precipitating factor such as recent antibiotic therapy and Jane should see her doctor for further investigation.

The doctor's view

Helen Jones should be advised to take Jane to the doctor. The description is certainly suggestive of oral thrush. If there were any doubt as to the diagnosis a swab could be taken for laboratory examination. If Jane did have thrush then treatment such as *miconazole oral gel* or *nystatin oral suspension* might be prescribed. Treatment is enhanced by cleaning the white plaques off with a cotton bud prior to application.

The next concern would be to determine a precipitating cause. General enquiries about Jane's health would be necessary. The doctor would be in a good position to know of previous medical history including any transfusions and family history. A general physical examination would be carried out, looking in particular for signs of anaemia, any rashes or bruising, enlargement of lymph nodes (glands), enlargement of abdominal organs (e.g. liver or spleen) or any other masses. The doctor would be looking for signs of a malignancy such as leukaemia or lymphoma. Almost certainly blood tests would be arranged. The doctor would also make an assessment of any HIV risk factors and counsel Helen and Jane accordingly before initiating any further action.

Case 2

A young mother asks for something to treat her baby son's mouth. You look inside the baby's mouth and see white patches on the tongue and inside the cheeks. The baby is 8 weeks old and has had the patches for 2 days: at first his mother thought they were milk curds. He had some antibiotic syrup last week for a chest infection and finished taking it yesterday. The baby is not taking any other medicines and his mother has not given him anything to treat the symptoms yet. He has no other symptoms.

The pharmacist's view

You could recommend the use of *miconazole oral gel* for this baby. He has a thrush infection following antiobiotic therapy which should respond well to the imidazole antifungal. His mother should use 2.5 ml of gel twice daily after feeds, applying it to the inside of the mouth and tongue. Treatment should be continued for 2 days after the problem has cleared up. If the symptoms have not gone after a week, the baby should be seen by the doctor.

The doctor's view

Oral thrush sounds the most likely diagnosis. It would be reasonable for the pharmacist to institute treatment in view of the baby's age alone, although in this case antibiotic treatment is an additional precipitating factor. If there was any doubt as to the diagnosis his mother could seek the advice of the health visitor. It might be useful to ask the mother whether or not she was breast feeding in case any gel needed applying to the nipples. When applying the gel to the mouth the plaques should be scraped off, if possible, to increase the effectiveness of the treatment.

Other Conditions

Insomnia

An estimated 8 million people in the UK have problems sleeping. Temporary insomnia is common and can often be managed by the pharmacist. The key to restoring appropriate sleep patterns is advice on sleep hygiene. Over-the-counter (OTC) products to aid sleep (the antihistamines *diphenhydramine* and *promethazine*) can help during the transition period and can also be useful in periodic and transient sleep problems. However, these products are advertised direct to the public and pharmacists report difficulties in declining sales for continued use. An initial focus on sleep hygiene and careful explanation that antihistamines are for short-term use are therefore important.

What you need to know
Age
Symptoms
Difficulty falling asleep
Waking during the night
Early morning waking
Poor sleep quality
Snoring
Duration
Previous history
Previous episodes
Contributory factors
Shift working, being away from home
Current sleep hygiene
Medication

Significance of questions and answers

Age

In elderly people the total duration of sleep is shorter and there is less deep stage 4 sleep. Nocturnal waking is more likely because sleep is generally more shallow. However, the person may still feel that they need more sleep and wish to take a medicine to help them sleep. Elderly people may nap during the day and this reduces their sleep need at night even further.

Many babies, toddlers and infants have poor sleep patterns which understandably can cause anxiety to parents. In these situations referral to the health visitor or doctor can be helpful. There are also some helpful self-help books and pamphlets available.

Symptoms
It is important to differentiate between the different types of sleep problems:
difficulty in falling asleep (sleep latency insomnia)
waking during the night
early morning waking
poor sleep quality
snoring.

Depression is an important cause of insomnia. Early morning waking is a classic symptom of depression. Here the patient may describe no problems in getting to sleep but waking in the early hours and not being able to get back to sleep. This pattern requires referral to the doctor for further investigation.

Duration
Sleep disorders are classified as:
transient (days)
short-term (up to 3 weeks)
chronic (longer than 3 weeks).
All chronic cases should be referred to the doctor.

Previous history
It is worth asking whether this is the first time problems in sleeping have occurred or whether there is a previous history. Where there is a previous history it is helpful to know what treatments have been tried. It is also useful to be aware of a history of depression or anxiety or some other mental illness.

Contributory factors
1 Shift work with changing shifts is a classic cause of sleep problems. Those who work away from home may experience difficulty in getting a good night's sleep because of the combination of travelling and staying in unfamiliar places.
2 Alcohol—while one or two drinks can help by decreasing sleep latency, the sleep cycle is disturbed by heavy or continuous alcohol consumption.
3 Life changes can cause disrupted sleep, for example, change or loss of job, moving house, bereavement, loss or separation, or the 'change of life' (i.e. menopause).
4 Other stressful life events might include exams, job interviews, celebrations (e.g. Christmas) and relationship difficulties.

Current sleep hygiene

It is worth asking about the factors known to contribute to effective sleep hygiene (see *Practical points*, below).

Medication

Some drugs can cause or contribute to insomnia including decongestants, *fluoxetine*, monoamine oxidase inhibitors (MAOIs), corticosteroids, appetite suppressants, *phenytoin* and *theophylline*. Medical problems can be associated with insomnia through pain (e.g. angina, arthritis, cancer and gastro-oesophageal reflux) or breathing difficulties (e.g. heart failure, chronic obstructive airways disease and asthma). Other medical conditions such as hyperthyroidism and Parkinson's disease can also cause insomnia.

> **When to refer**
>
> Suspected depression
> Chronic problem (longer than 3 weeks' duration)
> Children aged under 16

Treatment timescale

There should be an improvement within days: refer after a week if the problem is not resolved.

Management

Antihistamines (diphenhydramine, promethazine)

Antihistamines reduce sleep latency (the time taken to fall asleep) and also reduce nocturnal waking. They should be taken 20–30 minutes before bedtime and can be recommended for adults and children over 16 years old. Tolerance to their effects can develop and they should not be used for longer than 7–10 consecutive nights. *Diphenhydramine* has a shorter half-life than *promethazine*. Following a 50 mg dose of *diphenhydramine* there is significant drowsiness for 3–6 hours. These antihistamines have anticholinergic side effects including dry mouth and throat, constipation, blurred vision and tinnitus. These effects will be enhanced if the patient is taking another drug with anticholinergic effects (e.g. tricyclic antidepressants, phenothiazines—patients taking these drugs would be better referred anyway). Prostatic hypertrophy and closed-angle glaucoma are contra-indications to the use of *diphenhydramine* and *promethazine*. *Diphenhydramine* and *promethazine* should not be recommended for pregnant or breastfeeding women.

Benzodiazepines

Despite the UK Committee on Safety of Medicines statement on the use of benzodiazepines, recommending that these drugs are for short-term use only and should not be used for longer than 3 weeks, pharmacists are well aware that patients continue to be on these drugs for long periods of time. Research shows that success rates in weaning patients off benzodiazepines can be high. This is an area where pharmacists and doctors can work together and discussions with local doctors can initiate this process.

Complementary therapies

Some patients prefer 'alternative' treatments for insomnia, perceiving them as more 'natural'. Herbal remedies have been traditionally used for insomnia with valerian and hops the most commonly used ingredients. They are not recommended for pregnant or breastfeeding women. There are no reports of side effects.

Aromatherapy

Aromatherapy is effective in aiding relaxation. *Lavender oil* in particular has been shown to induce a sense of relaxation, as has *camomile*. One or 2 drops of the essential oil sprinkled on a pillow, or 3–4 drops in a warm (not hot) bath can be recommended.

Melatonin

Melatonin is currently only available on prescription in this country, however, it is widely used in the USA to treat insomnia. Melatonin is produced by the body's pineal gland during darkness and is thought to regulate sleep. Studies have shown that melatonin levels are lower in the elderly. Supplementation with melatonin can raise levels and help restore the sleep pattern. Melatonin has a short half-life (2–3 hours) and is subject to first-pass metabolism. Sub-lingual, controlled release products are therefore popular in the USA.

Nasal plasters for snoring

These adhesive nasal strips work by opening the nostrils wider and enabling the body to become accustomed to breathing through the nose rather than the mouth. A plaster is applied each night for up to a week to retrain the breathing process. The strips have been suggested for use in night-time nasal congestion during pregnancy.

Practical points

Sleep hygiene

Key points are:

establish a regular bedtime and waking time

consciously create a relaxation period before bedtime

no meals just before bed

no naps during the daytime

no caffeine after lunchtime

reduce extraneous noise (use earplugs if necessary)

get up if you can't sleep—go back to bed when you feel 'sleepy tired'

restrict alcohol intake to 1–2 units a day

restrict nicotine intake immediately before bedtime.

Bathing

A warm bath 1–2 hours (not immediately before) bedtime can help induce sleep.

Using heat

An electric blanket can help sleep by relaxing the muscles and increasing brain temperature. The effect is not needed throughout the night, only in inducing sleep. Using a timer to switch off the blanket after an hour or two is sensible.

Caffeine

The stimulant effect of caffeine in coffee, tea and cola drinks is considerable. Avoiding caffeine in the afternoon and evening is sensible advice.

Insomnia in practice

Case 1

Chris Jenkins, a 20-year-old student, comes into the pharmacy requesting some tablets to help him sleep. He says that he has had problems sleeping ever since returning from Indonesia 10 days ago. He says that he cannot get off to sleep because he does not feel tired. When he eventually does fall asleep, he sleeps fitfully and finds it difficult to get up in the morning. He has never suffered from insomnia before. He is otherwise well, is not taking any medicines and does not have any other problems or difficulties.

The pharmacist's view

Long-haul travel can result in disruption of the sleep pattern and some people are more affected by it than others. It would be reasonable to recommend that Chris takes an antihistamine (*diphenhydramine* or *promethazine*) for 4–5 days until the problem resolves. An alternative would be one of the herbal products to aid sleep. He should find that his normal sleep pattern is re-established within a week.

The doctor's view

This is quite likely to be a short-term problem due to his recent travelling. A very short course of antihistamines seems sensible to re-establish a better pattern. Many people who complain of insomnia do not always admit to other problems in their lives. It is therefore important to be alert to this possibility. If his insomnia does not resolve quickly, or if the pharmacist were to notice that Chris seemed low or anxious, a referral would be appropriate.

Case 2

Maureen Thomas, aged about 50, comes in asking for something to help her sleep. She says she has seen an advertisement for some tablets that will help. Maureen explains her sleep has been bad ever since she had her children, but over the last week it has got worse. She says she has had problems in getting off to sleep and recently has been waking early and not getting back to sleep. She says that she has had some worries at work and her Mum has been unwell… 'but that's all, no more than usual. I've had to put up with a lot worse and managed! I just need a few days good sleep and I'll be OK'. Otherwise she reveals that she is not on any other medication and has never troubled anyone before with her sleeping problem.

The pharmacist's view

This patient is experiencing a number of sources of stress and difficulty which are likely to be contributing to her sleep problems. In addition to having trouble getting to sleep, she is also waking early and unable to get back to sleep, indicating that the sleep disturbance is extensive. Early waking can also be a symptom of depression. It would be best for her to see the doctor and this will need a careful, persuasive explanation from the pharmacist. It would also be useful to talk about sleep hygiene to see if there are any practical actions that she could take to alleviate the problem. While the use of an antihistamine or herbal medicine for a few days would not be harmful, it may prevent her from seeking advice from the doctor. Therefore it would be better not to recommend a medicine on this occasion.

The doctor's view

Ideally this woman should be advised to make an appointment to see her doctor. It is possible that she would be reluctant to do so, as she gives the impression that she thinks she should be able to cope and should not have to trouble anyone else with her problems. If the pharmacist could persuade her that it is completely acceptable to seek advice from her doctor, this would be the best course of action. She sounds depressed and it would be helpful for a doctor to make a full assessment. This would include how she is feeling, how her life is being affected and what other symptoms she may have. It may be that she is also distressed by changes associated with the menopause.

Just the ability to talk to a good attentive accepting listener can be very beneficial. She may benefit from seeing a counsellor which the doctor can arrange. If her symptoms are severe and if she agrees, she may benefit from antidepressant medication.

Appendix: Summary of symptoms for direct referral

Chest
Chest pain
Shortness of breath
Wheezing
Swollen ankles
Blood in sputum
Palpitations
Persistent cough
Whooping cough
Croup
Sputum mucoid, coloured

Gut
Difficulty with swallowing
Blood in vomit
Bloody diarrhoea
Vomiting with constipation
Weight loss
Sustained alteration in bowel habit

Eye
Painful red eye
Loss of vision
Double vision

Ear
Pain
Discharge
Deafness
Irritation
Tinnitus
Vertigo

Genito-urinary
Difficulty in passing urine
Blood in urine
Abdominal/loin/back pain with
  cystitis
Temperature with cystitis
Urethral discharge
Vaginal discharge
Vaginal bleeding in pregnancy

Other
Neck stiffness/rigidity with
  temperature
Vomiting (persistent)

Index

Hyoscine, 19, 68, 88, 89, 216
  contra-indication, 216
Hypertension, 16
  cough remedies, 25
  headache, 182
  sympathomimetics contra-indication, 18, 30
Hyperthyroidism, 18, 21, 30
Hyperventilation, 53, 54
Hypnotics, antihistamines interaction, 19, 30, 48

Ibuprofen, 5, 77, 183, 185–6, 195, 199, 215, 217
  caution, 186
  children, 185
  contra-indication, 186, 215
  hypersensitivity, 186
    aspirin cross-sensitivity, 186, 215
  interactions, 186
  topical, 197
  unwanted effects, 185–6, 215
Ice-pack treatment, 197–8
Icthammol, 233
Imidazoles, 146, 148, 218, 222–3, 225, 244
  sensitivity reactions, 223
Imipramine, 100
Immunocompromised patient
  candidal infection, 37, 260
  cold sores, 152
  warts/verrucae, 157
Immunosuppressive therapy, 37
  candidiasis association, 260
Impetigo, 151
Indigestion (dyspepsia), 74–83
  age, 75
  case examples, 81–4
  diet, 77
  duration, 75
  management, 78–81
    antacids, 78–80
    H$_2$ antagonists, 81
  medication use, 77–9
  previous history, 75
  referral to doctor, 75, 77, 78, 81, 82
  smoking habit, 77
  symptoms, 74–6
  treatment timescale, 78
Indomethacin, 77, 81
Infectious mononucleosis (glandular fever), 36, 37, 40
Infective diarrhoea, 103–5
Inflammatory bowel disease, 61
Inhalants, 20, 31
Inhalation devices, 33
Insecticide policy, 249–50
Insomnia, 267–73
  age, 267–8
  case examples, 271–3

contributory factors, 268
  duration, 268
  management, 269–70
    antihistamines, 269, 271, 272
    benzodiazepines, 270
    complementary therapies, 270
    melatonin, 270
    practical advice, 270–1
  medication use, 269
  previous history, 268
  referral to doctor, 269, 272–3
  sleep hygiene, 269, 270–1
  symptoms, 268
  treatment timescale, 269
Intracranial pressure elevation, 180, 182
Ipecacuanha, 29
Iritis, 230
Iron deficiency, 61
Iron preparations
  abdominal pain, 77
  antacid interactions, 77, 80
  constipation, 97
  diarrhoea, 106
Irritable bowel syndrome, 112–18
  abdominal pain, 76, 112, 113, 118
  age, 112–13
  aggravating factors, 114
  bloating, 113
  bowel habit disturbance, 113
  case examples, 117–18
  complementary therapies, 116
  diarrhoea, 103, 105
  diet, 116
  duration, 113
  management, 114–16
    antidiarrhoeals, 116
    antispasmodics, 114–15, 117
    bulking agents, 116
  medication use, 114
  previous history, 114
  referral to doctor, 112, 113, 114, 117, 118
  symptoms, 113
  treatment timescale, 114
Ischaemic heart disease, 68
Isosorbide dinitrate, 73
Ispaghula, 95–6, 116
Itraconazole, 80

Joint pain (arthralgia), 193, 200

Kaolin, 107–8
  skin protectors, 122
Kaolin and morphine mixture, 108, 109
Kaposi's varicelliform eruption (eczema herpeticum), 154
Keratolytics
  acne, 140
  benzoyl peroxide, 140–1